No Shortcuts

The 10 Non-Negotiables of Wellbeing

No Shortcuts

The 10 Non-Negotiables of Wellbeing

Oli Mittermaier, MS

Adam Tibble, MD

CIT Clinics Press

Second Edition

ISBN (paperback): 979-8-9961173-1-4

Published by CIT Clinics Press

Printed in the United States of America

Disclaimer: The information in this book is for general informational and educational purposes only. It is not medical advice and is not intended to substitute for professional medical advice, diagnosis, or treatment. Always seek the advice of your physician or other qualified health provider with any questions you may have regarding a medical condition. The authors and publisher disclaim any liability arising directly or indirectly from the use of this book.

For our patients,
who showed us what was missing.

And our staff,
for whom this is a calling.

A Note on the Cover

Look at the cover. Enter the labyrinth and trace your finger through it until you arrive at the middle.

Then trace your way back out.

It's a stylized version of the labyrinth set into the floor of Chartres Cathedral, in France, sometime around 1200. Pilgrims have walked it for eight hundred years.

For us, this labyrinth is not about organized religion. It is a representation of practice and commitment to a process. In that sense it does elicit a kind of faith and trust. It represents the journey that is at the heart of the human experience.

Importantly, a labyrinth is not a maze. A maze is a puzzle — it has dead ends, false turns, places where you can get lost. A labyrinth has only one path. You enter at the bottom, you walk, and eventually you reach the center. There are no shortcuts. You can't skip ahead. You can't take a clever route that gets you there faster than someone who started behind you. Walking it methodically and patiently is the entire point.

The medieval pilgrims who walked the Chartres labyrinth understood this. Many of them did so as a substitute for the journey to Jerusalem, which most could not afford. The walking *is* the practice. The act is a pilgrimage. There is no version of the experience that involves getting to the center any faster. There are no shortcuts.

That's the metaphor we want this book to begin with.

For nearly a decade, we have worked with patients who arrived at CIT Clinics looking for a shortcut. Most of them do not call it that — they call it Ketamine, or Spravato, or something different. And those treatments usually do exactly what they were supposed to do. The neurological window opens. The fixed narrative loosens. Hope, becomes available again.

And then most of them go home to a life that has no infrastructure to hold the hope they'd been given.

That's when we started keeping the list that became this book. Ten things that consistently appeared in the background of every patient who got better, and were conspicuously absent in every patient who didn't. Not diagnoses. Not protocols. Just the unglamorous infrastructure of being a human animal in the modern world: sleep, movement, food, your home, your people, your purpose, your contribution, your capacity for joy.

There are no shortcuts to any of them. There's only the path. The good news is that the path exists. It has been walked before. The trail is clearly marked. You can't get lost in a labyrinth — you can only stop walking.

Also notice that the path doesn't end at the center. It ends, and then you turn around, and you walk back out. The walking is not about arriving at the center. The journey is what changes the person who walks. And the changed person leaves the labyrinth and rejoins the world with a new perspective (and skills!).

The work this book describes is not work you do for yourself alone. The endpoint of recovering your sense of Self is not a private experience of simply feeling better. The endpoint is being well enough to be useful — to your Self, to your family, your community, your patients, your colleagues, the people who haven't yet entered the labyrinth and are still looking for access.

You're holding the book because something brought you here. Maybe you're in the middle of your own walk and the path got harder than you expected. Maybe you're between treatments and trying to figure out what to build with the window someone opened for you. Maybe you're a clinician who keeps watching the same window close on patients you've genuinely helped, and you suspect, the way we came to suspect, that the missing piece isn't more medicines or clinical work.

Whatever brought you here, the book begins with the same premise the labyrinth begins with: there's only one path, and that path is 'through'.

There are no shortcuts. There never were.

There *is* a path, however. That's the point of this book.

Oli & Adam

Introduction

The Skills Nobody Taught You

Dave had faithfully followed every step the mental health system had offered him. Two rounds of antidepressants. Years of therapy. A psychiatric hospitalization. Two residential treatment programs. By the time he came to CIT Clinics for Ketamine treatment, he had accumulated more clinical contact than most physicians accumulate in a decade of practice. And, he was still, in his own words, despondent.

The Ketamine sessions went well. The neurological windows opened the way they often do — a loosening of the fixed narrative, a brief and genuine softening of the suffering that had calcified around his identity. After the third session, he looked at me (Oli) and said something I've heard in different forms from many patients: "I can feel that it's possible. I feel more hopeful. And I'm scared I don't know how to sustain this."

A few months later, he called me in tears from his home in Michigan. "It's back. All the progress I made in California is gone. I want it to end. Can you please come and help me."

This was an entirely different kind of house call. I packed my bags and flew to Michigan. I committed to staying with him for a month.

Dave was in his mid-fifties, recently forced out of the financial firm he'd built over decades under circumstances that were still being litigated. He'd won a large settlement and retired — technically. What he'd actually done was stop. The days had no structure, no purpose, and no container. He drove his sports car too fast, drank expensive scotch in the evenings, and spent the in-between hours cycling through grievances about the people who'd wronged him. He was divorced, struggled with his teenage kids, and freshly out of a two-year on-and-off relationship that had finally ended for good. He had every resource and no infrastructure.

His house reflected it. Piles of laundry in every room. A refrigerator stocked with light beer and sugary electrolyte drinks. A kitchen sink full of dishes. Cabinets filled with unused china. A home office buried under unopened mail. There was a pool and a workout room with a huge TV for football games. It was October. Winter was coming fast and Dave felt grim.

We started small. Mornings began with a workout, followed by a cold plunge in the pool (Michigan in the Fall). We went to the grocery store together. I cooked and got him to help chop carrots. We sorted laundry, opened the mail, drove to his church to find whatever was left of his community. We got outside and walked. We played pickleball. In the evenings, he talked — mostly about the firm, the lawsuit, the ways he'd been wronged — and I listened, and we journaled, and sometimes we went back outside and got in the cold water again because it was the fastest reset for both of us.

By the end of the second week, something had shifted. Not dramatically. He was sleeping a little more consistently. He was eating food he'd contributed to cooking. He had somewhere to be in the morning.

That's when I understood what I was actually looking at.

The Ketamine had worked. The neuroplastic activation had begun. And yet, what Dave didn't have — what no one had thought to give him — was any infrastructure to climb through it. His days had no anchor. His body had no rhythm. His living space had no order. His world had no real people in it. The treatment was opening a window but the rest of his life remained closed.

I started keeping a different kind of list.

Not diagnoses or treatment protocols. A list of things that kept appearing in the background of every patient who was getting better — and conspicuously absent in every patient who wasn't. They weren't clinical findings. Nothing in the Diagnostic and Statistical Manual of Mental Disorders (DSM) covers "hasn't had a real conversation with another human being in four months." No Current Procedural Terminology (CPT)insurance code reimburses for "has been eating cereal over the sink since the breakup." But these things kept showing up with the reliability of a physical law, as the difference between a window that stayed open and one that quietly closed.

Over nearly a decade of working with depressed, anxious and despondent people, the list coalesced at ten non-negotiables.

A Peculiar Double Standard

You have probably seen many such videos on social media. A freestyle motocross rider launches off a ramp, detaches from the motorcycle mid-flight, performs two full rotations through space while the bike does its own separate acrobatics, then somehow reunites with the machine and lands — alive, smiling, enthusiastically pointing at the energy drink sponsor on his helmet.

Or consider a Navy pilot landing an F/A-18 on a carrier deck at night. Rain. Eight hours of mission fatigue. The deck is pitching in the open ocean. The entire landing strip is shorter than a city block. The margin for error is not small. It is zero.

Or watch a great stand-up comedian hold two thousand strangers in the palm of their hand for ninety minutes. The pause that lands in exactly the right place. The joke that arrives so naturally the audience gasps before they laugh. The way the whole thing feels like he just thought of it — like you're watching someone think out loud, brilliantly, in real time. What you're actually watching is the product of ten years of dying on stage in half-empty bars. Of driving four hours to do seven minutes for an audience of nine. The same joke told three hundred times in three hundred rooms until the word that wasn't quite right got replaced by the word that was. The pause that feels spontaneous has been placed in exactly that spot because he discovered — through repetition — that a half-second longer and the laugh is twice as big. This is the infrastructure that was built and practiced over years until it became invisible.

We recognize these as skills. It seems obvious to us that behind each of these extraordinary performances is an architecture of effort we haven't been privy to: the ten thousand repetitions, the coaches, the failures, the micro-adjustments, the years of showing up when it was anything but fun. Nobody watches a carrier landing and thinks he must have been born with the *land-jets-on-boats gene*. Nobody watches the comedian and thinks *he just has a natural gift for timing*.

And yet, when we encounter someone who moves through life with genuine grace and equanimity — not the Instagram kind, not the false brightness of someone performing for an audience, but actual, durable okayness with existence — something shifts in how we explain it. We don't think: ten thousand repetitions. We don't think: the coaches, therapy sessions, books, the failures, the years of showing up when it was painful and arduous.

We think: lucky.

We think: good genes.

We think: some mysterious disposition handed out at birth that the rest of us somehow missed.

We watch a person stay grounded when their life is falling apart and we call it grace, as if grace were a gift rather than a practice. We watch someone move through grief without being destroyed by it and we call them strong, as if strength were a trait rather than a skill built, slowly, from the wreckage of harder moments. We watch a person maintain genuine connection and warmth across decades of a marriage and we say they're just like that — as if that explained anything at all.

It's a peculiar double standard, and once you see it you can't unsee it.

Physical mastery? Obviously the product of effort. Psychological and emotional mastery? Apparently a matter of cosmic luck. The motocross rider *earned* his three seconds of airborne impossibility. The comedian *earned* her pause. But the person who has learned to regulate their nervous system, stay present under pressure, and build a life that actually feels worth living — somehow we assumed they were just born that way.

This is delusional, magical thinking and it simply isn't true.

We forget that the brain doesn't care what you're practicing. It is a prediction machine running on two basic principles: 1) neurons that fire together wire together, and 2) neurons that stop firing together unwire from one another.[1] Repeat something enough times over time, and it becomes automatic — because the structure and function of your brain, your nervous system, your whole organism adjusts itself to perform that specific skill. This works identically whether you're landing an aircraft on an aircraft carrier, playing violin for an auditorium of music aficionados, or keeping your cool when life goes sideways.

System 1 and System 2

Psychologist Daniel Kahneman describes two operating systems running in parallel inside your head.[2] System 1 is fast, automatic, and effortless — the part of you that drives a familiar route without thinking, flinches before you've registered the threat, or reaches for the phone before you've decided to. System 2, on the other hand, is slow, deliberate, and effortful — the part that does long division, weighs a difficult decision, or notices that you've been scrolling for forty minutes. Most of your life is run by System 1. System 2 mostly shows up to rationalize what System 1 already decided.[3]

Here's what that means in practice: the behaviors that shape your life most aren't the ones you think carefully about. They're the ones that have been handed off to System 1 — running automatically, below the level of deliberate choice, because you've done them enough times that your brain stopped asking permission. That handoff is neuroplasticity at work.

Neuroplasticity is agnostic. It doesn't moralize. It will faithfully wire up whatever you give it the most repetitions of (System 1) — whether that's equanimity or reactivity, presence or panic, self-regulation or impulsivity.

So here is the question that should probably keep us up at night: why do we treat the skills required to be a functional, resilient, connected adult human as if they were inherited traits rather than trainable capacities?

Nobody wakes up able to land a jet on a moving ship. Why would anyone wake up knowing how to regulate their nervous system, maintain a decades-long friendship, or stay grounded when life goes sideways?

We literally are what we repeatedly do. This isn't a bumper sticker. It's a description of how our neurobiology works.

The Ten Non-Negotiables

After thousands of hours working with people in psychological crisis we have observed that the factors that most reliably predict whether someone actually gets better — not just stabilized, not just managed, but genuinely recovers and is able to build a life that feels worth living — isn't in the typical psychiatric treatment plan. There is no ICD-10 entry for 'can't locate important documents in their apartment.' Insurance doesn't reimburse for 'hasn't tackled the pile of laundry since the breakup.'

These things exist in some parallel universe that apparently doesn't count as real mental health — even though, neurobiologically speaking, they absolutely do.

True, the credit card debt didn't *cause* the depression in any strict clinical sense. But try climbing out of a depressive episode while creditors are calling and your prefrontal cortex is running on 'constant low-grade financial terror.' The same goes for a living space that is cluttered and in chronic disarray. Or sleep that comes in fragments. Or months without feeling like you've contributed anything meaningful to another human being.

These aren't the *causes* of mental illness per se. They're the friction points — the places where the demands of being a mammal in the modern world grind against a brain that evolved for a very different environment. This friction, left unaddressed, becomes emotional and spiritual burnout. Chronic friction leads to damage. Small problems compound into large ones.

The Natural World

For roughly 300,000 years, Homo sapiens lived in direct, daily contact with the natural world. Not as weekend recreation. As the entire context of existence. We woke with the light. We walked on uneven ground. We navigated by landmarks rather than screens. We ate food that came from soil. We smelled rain, soil, and wood smoke. Our nervous systems were not built in offices, apartments, or climate-controlled cars. They were built in forests, on plains, near water, under open sky. The sensory inputs we now consider recreational extras — natural light, varied terrain, the smell of plants and soil, the sound of wind and moving water — were, for the vast majority of human history, simply what existence felt like.

Modern indoor life is, in evolutionary terms, a radical and very recent experiment. The average American now spends more than 90 percent of their time indoors.[43] We have swapped full-spectrum natural light for fluorescent overhead lighting. We have traded irregular, variable terrain for flat, climate-controlled floors. We have replaced the smells of forests and fields with processed air. Our nervous systems — still running the same underlying firmware they ran on the savanna — are making do in an environment they were not built for.

The research on what happens when we reintroduce regular contact with natural environments is consistent and, when you understand the evolutionary context, entirely unsurprising. Spending time in natural settings measurably reduces cortisol, lowers blood pressure, and restores the directed-attention capacity that modern cognitive work relentlessly depletes.[44] Exposure to natural light anchors the circadian system that governs sleep, mood, and hormonal regulation.[45] The microbiome — increasingly understood as a central player in mood and immune function — is meaningfully shaped by contact with soil and natural environments.[46] Even brief exposure to trees, water, and open sky triggers a shift in the autonomic nervous system, from the sympathetic vigilance state that indoor environments tend to sustain, toward the parasympathetic recovery state where actual restoration happens.[47]

This isn't a case for abandoning modernity. It's a case for recognizing that the friction you feel — the low-grade fatigue, the restlessness, the sense of something missing that no productivity system quite addresses — may be, in part, the friction of an organism living out or sync from the environment it was built for. You are not broken. You are simply a biological system running in conditions it wasn't designed to run in, without the environmental inputs it was designed to receive.

You'll find the natural world threaded throughout this book — not as a chapter, but as a constant. Because the same way a leaky roof affects every room in the house, chronic disconnection from the natural environment affects every one of the ten non-negotiables. It shows up in sleep, movement, self-care, quality of relationships, capacity for joy and awe. It is one of the easiest and most underrated adjustments available, and best of all, it usually costs nothing.

Going outside is not a lifestyle preference. It is a biological requirement that most of us have quietly stopped meeting.

The Rule of 60

There's a principle in aviation called the Rule of 60. For every one degree a plane drifts off course, it will miss its destination by one mile for every 60 miles flown. On a short flight, one degree is a rounding error. On a flight from San Francisco to New York, that same one degree puts you down in a field in New Jersey. Small errors compounded over time have catastrophic consequences.

The ten non-negotiables work the same way. Not dramatic failures — incremental degrees that compound over time. A sleep schedule that slips by thirty minutes. A week without meaningful contact with another person. A month of meals that arrive in frozen cardboard boxes. None of it feels like a monumental decision. But the math catches up. And by the time it does, System 1 — the fast, automatic part of the brain that runs on habit — has already made the call, long before System 2 — the slower, effortful part that weighs consequences — gets a vote.

This is the unsexy truth about well-being: it runs on infrastructure. Not inspiration. Not insight. **Infrastructure!**

After nearly a decade, the infrastructure that mattered most consistently stabilized at ten domains. I've come to think of them as the Ten Non-Negotiables — not because they are ten equally weighted pillars, but because chronic depletion in any one of them creates a drag on the entire system that makes everything else harder.

Foundation — Your Biological Base

- **Sleep** — The bedrock. Compromise this and every other system degrades.
- **Movement** — The signal that tells every system in your body to grow stronger and adapt.
- **Nutrition & Hydration —** The raw materials your neurochemistry runs on. Garbage in, garbage out.

Structure — Your Stability Systems

- **Self-Care** — The ongoing practice of keeping your window of tolerance open rather than waiting for it to close.
- **Physical Environment** — The spaces you inhabit shape your nervous system's baseline, below the level of conscious awareness.
- **Life Administration** — The unglamorous scaffolding that, when solid, is invisible — and when neglected, is all you can see.

Thriving — A Life Worth Living

- **Community & Belonging** — Humans are obligately social. Isolation is a physiological stressor, not just a feeling.
- **Meaning & Purpose** — The compass that makes the daily navigation make sense.
- **Being of Service** — Meaning doesn't come from thinking about yourself. It comes from being useful to others.
- **Joy, Play & Awe** — Not optional. The neurochemical regulators that keep the entire system from collapsing into gray.

The ten non-negotiables are skills — trainable, measurable, improvable capacities. They are not things you are either born with or without and therefore fixed and immutable. The brain that struggles with sleep hygiene or social connection today is the same brain that can get measurably better at both through the right kind of repetition and support. That's not optimism. That's neuroplasticity.

You don't need to be perfect at any of them. You just need to be good enough that chronic depletion in one domain isn't continuously undermining the other nine. The goal is a functional floor — not an optimized ceiling.

Building Your House

Imagine building a house that represents your life. You want safety, stability, warmth, beauty — all of it. But before any of that is possible, certain things are non-negotiable regardless of your preferences. The foundation has to be poured before the walls go up. The walls have to be sound before you hang anything on them. You cannot host an enjoyable dinner party for your friends in a house if the roof is leaking and the floor is collapsing.

The three tiers of the ten non-negotiables follow the same logic.

The Foundation is biological. Sleep, movement, and nutrition are the concrete and steel on which everything else rests. If this tier is chronically compromised, the entire structure above it is unstable regardless of how much effort you put into the floors above.

The Structure is your stability system. Self-care, physical environment, and effective life administration are the walls and systems that protect you from the elements — the window of tolerance kept open, the space that supports rather than undermines, the scaffolding that keeps obligations from becoming crises. A solid foundation with no walls still leaves you exposed.

The Thriving tier is what makes the house a home. Community, service, purpose, joy — these are the warmth, the guests, the light in the windows. But they cannot be built and sustained on a foundation that isn't solid or walls that are caving in.

The Golden Rule of Construction: when you feel stuck at a higher tier — when you can't find your purpose, can't build community, can't access joy — the solution is always found one tier down. Fix the wall before you hang the painting. Fix the floor before you fix the wall.

How This Process Works

Each of the ten chapters that follow is structured the same way. You'll meet a person whose life in that domain has collapsed or stalled in a recognizable way. You'll read the science that explains why — the mechanism, not just the prescription. You'll find a self-assessment quiz to locate yourself honestly within that domain. And then you'll move into the practice: how to build the skill and desirable habit, how to make the changes stick, and how to commit to something specific before you turn the page.

The Four Drivers Of Behavior Change

The practice section of each chapter is built around four principles that appear consistently across all ten non-negotiables. I call them the Four Drivers of Behavior Change. You don't need to understand them fully before you begin — they'll become familiar through repetition, the same way any skill does. But here is the short version:

1. Start Small

The fastest way to fail at behavior change is to attempt too much at once. System 1 — your fast, automatic, habit-running brain — treats large changes as threats and mobilizes resistance accordingly. Starting embarrassingly small bypasses that resistance entirely. One rep. One minute. One thing. The goal isn't to be impressive. The goal is to get the first rep done.

2. Shape Your Environment

Your environment makes most of your decisions before you're consciously aware a decision is being made. Willpower is a finite and unreliable resource. Environmental design is permanent and free. Make the right behavior the easiest behavior and let the architecture do the work your motivation can't sustain.

3. Link Habits

New behaviors don't survive on their own. They need to be anchored to something that already runs automatically. 'After I brush my teeth, I will...' is not a trick — it's implementation intention science.[4] You're attaching a new behavior to an existing neural highway rather than trying to carve a new road through sheer willpower.

4. Celebrate Wins

The moment immediately following a new behavior is the neurological window in which the habit circuit either strengthens or stalls. A genuine internal acknowledgment — 'good,' said and meant — fires the same dopaminergic signal as external praise.[5] Skip it and you're leaving your most powerful reinforcement mechanism unused.

These four principles are the same ones BJ Fogg, James Clear, and decades of behavioral science have arrived at through different routes.[6] They appear in every chapter not because they are repeated for emphasis but because they genuinely apply to every domain. The mechanism is the same whether you're building a sleep habit or a service practice. The brain doesn't care what you're wiring. It cares that you repeat it under conditions that make repetition likely.

How to Use This Book

You can read this book straight through or navigate by need. If you're in the middle of a crisis and sleep is the first thing to go, start with chapter one. If your foundation is reasonably stable but your life feels hollow and purposeless, start with chapter nine. The tier model in the conclusion will help you triage if you're unsure.

I strongly recommend against trying to work all ten chapters simultaneously. The research on behavior change is clear: attempting multiple changes at once increases cognitive load, depletes motivation, and reduces the probability that any of the changes will stick. Pick one chapter. Work it until the commitment page feels like a description of who you are rather than a prescription for who you should become. Then pick the next one.

Each chapter ends with a commitment page — four fields: a specific new behavior, an environmental setup, a trigger, and a celebration. These are not aspirations. They are implementation intentions — the specific format that behavioral research shows most reliably converts intention into action.[7] Fill them in. The more specific you are, the more likely the behavior is to stick.

The quiz at the start of each chapter is a tool, not a judgment. Answer honestly. This is for your eyes only. The score tells you where you are, not who you are. It's a snapshot, not a sentence.

Establishing Your Baseline

Before you read the first chapter, take ten minutes with these questions. Write the answers down. Not because someone will check them, but because the act of writing activates a different kind of knowing than the act of reading. This is your baseline — the before picture. We'll come back to it frequently as you work your process.

1. **If you could change three things about your daily life overnight, what would they be?**

2. **Name three patterns, habits, or beliefs that you know are holding you back.**

3. **What has been your biggest personal success? How did you achieve it? Who helped you?**

4. **Describe your life as you want it to be in five years. Write it in the present tense, as if it is already true.**

5. **Name three behaviors you believe would improve your life if you did them consistently. What has stopped you so far?**

6. **In two months, how will you know if this has been worth the effort? What will be different?**

You have the answers. What you may not yet have is the infrastructure to act on them consistently. That's what the next ten chapters are for.

The people you're about to meet — Beth, Marcus, Mark, Lusia, Arthur, Melanie, Daniel, Jennifer, Paul, Bruno — are composites drawn from real clinical experience. Their struggles are specific and their first steps are surprisingly small. That's the point.

None of them did anything extraordinary. But, all of them did something real. Something actionable.

That underappreciated distinction is the point of this book..

Sleep

Skill #1: Building The Foundation

"The best bridge between despair and hope is a good night's sleep."
— E. Joseph Cossman

Beth

Beth was 38, recently divorced, juggling two kids, a full-time job, and the kind of stress that had calcified her shoulders into stone. There was no off switch. Only the next thing, and the thing after that, and the quietly growing suspicion that this was simply what her life had become and would always be.

Nights were the hardest. After the homework battles and the dishes and the relentless noise of her own thoughts, she'd finally collapse into bed — only to lie there in the blue glow of her phone, scrolling through other people's seemingly happier lives until midnight. Vacations she wasn't taking. Couples who looked easy together. She knew Instagram was a highlight reel edited by wishful thinking and anxiety. She scrolled anyway.

Morning arrived like punishment. Foggy. Irritable. Caffeine delivered intravenously just to get out the door. She'd snap at one of the kids over something small — a spilled cup, a lost shoe — and spend the commute marinating in guilt about it.

She told herself this was just what life looked like now. Exhaustion was the tax you paid for surviving a divorce. But when even her weekends felt like wading through wet cement — forgetting basic tasks, crying in the car without knowing why — Beth realized something she hadn't wanted to admit. She wasn't just tired. She was unraveling.

One evening, after a meltdown over bedtime chaos that left everyone in tears including her, she sat on the cold floor of her bedroom and made a promise. Small and unglamorous and entirely private: no more phone in bed. That was it. That was the whole plan.

It felt almost too small to matter.

But that first night, after ten quiet minutes with a paperback she'd bought months ago and never opened, her eyelids grew heavy. She fell asleep before finishing the chapter.

The next morning wasn't miraculous. She was still tired. But there was a trace of clarity she hadn't felt in months — like a window cracked open in a room sealed all winter.

She built on it. Lights dimmed an hour before bed. A walk with the kids after dinner. Herbal tea instead of wine. Slowly the nights stretched longer and deeper, and the mornings felt less like punishment and more like a beginning.

Beth stopped thinking of sleep as something stolen from her. It became a practice. An anchor. And over time, an identity: she was no longer barely holding it together. She was a rested mother — with enough left in the tank to actually show up for the people who needed her most.

Sleep Quiz

Before we get into specifics, take two minutes to answer these questions. Answer honestly so you get a sense of how this past week has actually been for you.

Overall, how would you rate your sleep this past week?

⓪ Very unsatisfying ① Unsatisfying ② Fairly satisfying ③ Very satisfying

On average, how rested did you feel in the mornings?

⓪ Very unrested ① Somewhat unrested ② Fairly rested ③ Very rested

How many nights did you wake up one or more times?

⓪ Every night ① Most nights ② A few nights ③ Not once

How often did you take a sleeping aid?

⓪ Every night ① Most nights ② A few nights ③ Never

How often did you need caffeine or stimulants to become alert?

⓪ Every day ① Most days ② A few days ③ Never

Your Score: __________ (Total: 0–15)

- If 0–5: Start with one small, consistent change to your bedtime routine.
- If 6–10: Refine habits and remove your key sleep disruptors.
- If 11–15: Maintain and optimize for deeper, more restorative rest.

What Sleep Is

Sleep is not a luxury. It's not something you earn by being productive enough during the day, or something you can borrow against and pay back on weekends. Sleep is a non-negotiable operating requirement — a complex, active process in which your body and mind temporarily disconnect from the external world to perform maintenance that simply cannot be done while you're awake.

Your body is designed to spend nearly a third of its existence in this state. Evolution is not sentimental. It doesn't preserve behaviors that don't serve survival. The fact that every mammal on Earth sleeps — even though sleep leaves them acutely vulnerable to predation — is the clearest possible signal that whatever happens during those hours is worth the risk.

Here's what's actually happening while you're unconscious:

Your brain is clearing out metabolic waste through the glymphatic system — a literal nightly detox that protects your long-term neurological health[8]. It's consolidating memories, pruning unnecessary neural connections, and processing the emotional residue of your day. Your immune system is restoring its defenses. Your body is repairing tissue and recalibrating hormones. You are not 'doing nothing.' You are running one of the most sophisticated repair and optimization protocols in the known biological universe.

The Two Systems That Control Sleep

Two biological systems govern when you sleep and when you don't[9]:

The first is your **Circadian Rhythm** — the internal 24-hour clock that regulates your body's timing across virtually every organ system. It's set primarily by light. Morning light triggers a cortisol spike that shifts you toward alertness. Darkness cues the release of melatonin, signaling that it's time to power down. This is the same ancient system that once prevented your ancestors from wandering into lion territory after dark. Now it mostly keeps you from answering work emails at 3 a.m. — or should.

The second is **Sleep Pressure**, technically called homeostatic sleep drive. The longer you're awake, the more adenosine — a byproduct of neuronal activity — accumulates in your brain[10]. Think of it as biochemical sediment building up in a clear pool. Sleep flushes it out. Caffeine, for the record, doesn't remove the adenosine. It blocks the receptors that detect it.[11] The sediment keeps accumulating. When the caffeine clears, the full weight of built-up sleep pressure comes crashing down — which is why that afternoon energy crash hits like an avalanche.

Through the night, your brain cycles between Non-REM and REM sleep in roughly 90-minute loops.[12] Non-REM is deep maintenance mode: tissue repair, immune function upgrades, memory consolidation. REM sleep is where the more interesting work happens — emotional processing, creative integration, and that nightly flush of metabolic waste. Dreams, when they occur, are a byproduct of the brain running its cleanup routines with the sensory inputs turned off. Occasionally the results are bizarre. This is normal.

Why Sleep Is a Hub, Not Just a Spoke

Degrade sleep from the equation and the whole system falls apart. Not slowly, not eventually — pretty much immediately.

A single night of poor sleep impairs reaction time, working memory, and emotional regulation to a measurable degree. Miss 24 hours, and your cognitive performance mimics a blood-alcohol level of 0.10%[13] — legally impaired in every U.S. state. Your brain shifts into what cognitive scientists call System 1 dominance: fast, reflexive, impulsive. The slower, more deliberate System 2 — the part that plans, pauses, evaluates consequences, and resists the third slice of cake — starts running on fumes.

The Cost of Neglect

- Irritability and low frustration tolerance: Every slow driver feels like a personal insult. Every minor inconvenience becomes a potential confrontation.
- Brain fog and poor decision-making: A sleep-deprived System 2 isn't just slower — it's unreliable. You're making choices from a compromised instrument.
- Increased cravings for sugar and stimulants: A drowsy prefrontal cortex loses control over reward circuits. Caffeine and sugar stop being vices and start feeling like survival strategies.
- Lower motivation and productivity: System 2's drive falters. System 1 coasts toward comfort and avoidance.
- 'Tired but wired' at night: A dysregulated circadian rhythm keeps stress hormones elevated — exhausted all day, unable to wind down at night.

The Benefits of Consistent, Quality Sleep

- Consistent energy and mental clarity: System 1 and System 2 stop competing for cognitive resources.
- Emotional balance and resilience: Amygdala reactivity decreases. You stop reacting and start responding.
- Stronger immunity and faster physical recovery: Your body runs its maintenance cycles without interruption.
- Sharper memory, focus, and creativity: System 2 has the bandwidth to connect disparate ideas, solve problems, and retain what you learn.

- More patience and presence: You show up differently — to your kids, your partner, your work — when you're not running on a depleted system.

Sleep and Long-Term Mental Health

There's a bidirectional relationship between sleep and mental health that's worth being precise about: poor sleep doesn't just make you feel emotionally worse — it actively creates and sustains the neurological conditions for mood disorders to take hold and persist.

During deep non-REM sleep, your brain prunes unused neural connections and consolidates the ones tied to new learning and memory.[14] During REM, it processes the emotional residue of your waking hours — essentially running the day's experiences through an integration algorithm that reduces their charge and converts them into usable knowledge. Deprive the brain of this process consistently, and the emotional backlog accumulates. Reactivity rises. The threshold for overwhelm lowers. Depression and anxiety find easier purchase.

Here's the vicious loop: poor sleep worsens mood. Worsened mood disrupts sleep.[15] A dysregulated nervous system — System 1 running hot and paranoid, System 2 sluggish and overwhelmed — becomes the new default. You're more reactive, less reflective, and making decisions from an instrument that's been degraded by the very thing it most needs.

Protecting sleep is not an act of self-indulgence. It's the most foundational form of mental health maintenance available to you — and it's free.

How to Build Sleep Skills

Knowing that sleep matters isn't the same as sleeping well. The science you just read is necessary — but information without behavior change is just expensive trivia. What follows is how you build the actual skill.

Sleep hygiene is practiced, not acquired. You get better at it the same way you get better at anything: specific goals, deliberate practice, real feedback, and incremental challenge. Here's how that maps onto your actual life.

Start Small

- Get two minutes of natural light within 30–60 minutes of waking. Step outside if you can — a doorstep, a balcony, even a short walk down the driveway. If that's not possible, stand at a window with direct daylight rather than interior light. This is not ambiance. Natural light — full-spectrum, even on an overcast day — is approximately ten times stronger than indoor artificial light and is the primary signal your suprachiasmatic nucleus uses to set your circadian clock for the next 24 hours.[48] A reliable morning light signal in the morning means a stronger melatonin signal at night, which means deeper sleep, easier waking, and more consistent mood across the day. The entire downstream effect starts here. Two minutes. Outside.

- Shift your bedtime 5 minutes earlier this week. Not 30 minutes. Not an hour. Five. Add another 5 next week. Let the nervous system adapt rather than rebel.

- Track one pre-bed habit before trying to overhaul everything. One variable. One data point. Build from there.

Shape Your Environment

Willpower is a finite, unreliable resource. Environment is permanent and free. Design the room to do the work your willpower can't sustain.

- Dim lights and switch to warm tones 90 minutes before bed. Put it on a timer so the decision is already made.
- Charge your phone outside the bedroom. Not on silent. Not face-down. Outside. Remove the temptation entirely rather than trying to resist it.
- Keep a book you actually enjoy on your nightstand. Replace the default behavior (scroll) with an alternative that's already there.

Link Habits

You already have established routines. Use them as anchors. The goal is to let System 1 — your habit brain — take over from System 2 so that your sleep routine runs on autopilot instead of willpower.

- 'After I brush my teeth, I will take 10 intentional slow breaths to center myself.' The dental routine already fires automatically. Attach the new behavior and it inherits some of that automaticity.
- Pair breathwork — a physiological sigh (double inhale through the nose, long exhale through the mouth) — with turning off the last light. Body and brain get the signal simultaneously.
- Use the 5-4-3-2-1 countdown to shut down screens when the 'one more episode' loop starts. Interrupt the pattern before it completes.
- Move your morning light exposure outside by (coffee on the doorstep, a 5-minute walk before anything else, opening the back door and standing in it) immediately after getting up. The light is the anchor. Everything else catches a ride.

Celebrate the Wins

Celebration isn't optional sentimentality. It's the dopaminergic signal that tells your brain this behavior is worth repeating. Skip it and you're leaving the most powerful reinforcement mechanism in your neurological arsenal unused.

- After your bedtime routine, pause and acknowledge it. A genuine 'good' — said aloud or internally — fires the same reward circuits as external praise. Use them.
- Keep a simple sleep log. Mark your streaks. Visible progress activates the completion drive — the same mechanism that makes you want to finish a nearly-full stamp card.
- Treat each night as a practice rep. Not a test you pass or fail — a rep that builds the circuit. Some reps are better than others. All of them count.

Your Action Steps

1. Start Small

The goal is to make the habit feel impossible to fail:

- "On days when I have zero capacity for a full routine, the one thing I will do no matter what is ____________________ (e.g., put my phone on the charger, change into pajamas, turn off the overhead light)."
- "I will shift my bedtime earlier by ________ minutes this week — not 30, not an hour. Just ________ minutes."
- "If I can't sleep after ________ minutes, I will get out of bed rather than lie there fighting it."

2. Shape Your Environment

Design for the version of yourself who will be tired and low on willpower at 10 p.m.:

- "I will charge my phone in the __________________ (kitchen, hallway, bathroom) so it is not within reach in bed."
- "I will dim the lights in the __________________ at _______ PM using __________________ (a timer, a smart plug, a reminder on my phone)."
- "I will place __________________ on my pillow this morning so I have to physically move it before I can get into bed tonight."

3. Link Habits

Use what already runs on autopilot:

- "Immediately after brushing my teeth, I will __________________ (do three slow breaths, read one page, turn on the white noise machine)."
- "The moment I walk into my bedroom for the last time tonight, I will immediately __________________ (turn on the fan, put my phone in the drawer, close the blackout blinds)."
- "After I change into pajamas, I will signal that the day is finished by __________________ (saying 'shutdown complete,' doing a 60-second stretch, setting tomorrow's alarm)."

4. Celebrate the Wins

Reinforce the behavior so your brain wants to repeat it:

- "When I wake up feeling rested, I will take ten seconds to say to myself: ____________________ ('This is what happens when I take care of myself,' 'Good job.')."
- "I will track my progress by marking an X on ____________________ every morning I stick to my plan."
- "If I hit my lights-out time for 3 nights in a row, I will treat myself to ____________________."

My Sleep Commitment

Write it down. Specific. Simple. Small enough that you'll actually do it.

New Behavior:
What, specifically, will you do? (Keep it small.)

The Setup:
How will you prepare the environment for success?

The Trigger:
I will do this immediately before/after I:

The Celebration:
I will acknowledge my success by:

Becoming You

At first, sleep feels like a wish:

I should go to bed earlier. I should stop scrolling at night. I should finally wake up rested.

But 'should' rarely survives stress, busyness, or the gravitational pull of one more episode. Real rest doesn't arrive in occasional weekend marathons of catching up. It grows through repeated, ordinary, almost boring acts: turning off the screens ten minutes earlier, dimming the lights after dinner, stepping outside in the morning sun to remind your body it's time to be awake.

Each act strengthens the neural and hormonal circuits that regulate your rhythms and restore your mind. Over time, System 2 — the deliberate part of you that sets alarms, makes rules, and reminds you to put the phone down — begins to pass the baton to System 1. Sleep becomes less of a struggle and more of a reflex.

You stop seeing yourself as someone 'trying' to get good sleep. You start seeing yourself as a person who protects and values rest.

This shift is not cosmetic. You're no longer dragging yourself through the day on fumes, promising you'll catch up later. You become someone whose energy, mood, and clarity flow from a steady foundation of action-based recovery. Sleep ceases to be a fragile hope at the end of the day. It becomes part of who you are: a rested, present, resilient human being.

Beth got there by reading, creating a bed-time routine, drinking tea instead of wine. She took one step at a time. Not in a week. Not perfectly. But consistently enough that it changed everything else. So can you.

Movement

Skill #2: The Energy Multiplier

"If exercise could be packed into a pill, it would be the most widely prescribed and beneficial medicine in the nation."
— Dr. Robert Butler

"Exercise is the single most powerful tool you have to optimize your brain function."
— John Ratey

Marcus

Marcus was 44, a VP at a tech startup, and the kind of guy who used to play pickup basketball three times a week in college — the one who'd dive for loose balls, who'd stay an extra thirty minutes just to run one more set of sprints. Now his idea of movement was the walk from his car to the office. A hundred yards, maybe. Door to door.

Between back-to-back meetings that bled into each other like watercolors, his kids' schedules, and a marriage that required actual attention to stay healthy, the gym had become a relic. A dusty membership card in the back of his wallet. A direct debit he kept meaning to cancel. A source of the particular shame that lives not in failure but in the long, quiet avoidance of it.

He told himself he'd get back to it when things slowed down. Things never slowed down. They just changed shape.

Exercise wasn't joyful anymore. It was another item on a list of obligations he was silently failing — filed alongside flossing regularly and calling his father more often.

Then came the moment that cracked him open. A Sunday afternoon in the backyard, playing tag with his seven-year-old daughter. She was fast, delighted, completely feral in the way only small children can be. He lasted thirty seconds before his hands found his knees. Chest heaving. Vision slightly narrow at the edges. She stopped running and looked up at him with something uncomfortably close to concern. Dad, are you okay?

He laughed it off. But that night, alone with the truth in the way you can only be at 11pm when the house is quiet, he sat with what had happened. His body had become a stranger. Not an enemy — a stranger. Someone he used to know well, had lost touch with, and wasn't sure how to call.

The next morning, Marcus didn't go to the gym. He laced up a pair of running shoes he found at the back of the closet and walked around the block. One lap. Ten minutes. Nothing worthy of posting on social media. But entirely, uncomplicatedly his.

What he noticed, on that first lap and on the ones that followed, surprised him. Not the movement itself — he'd expected that to be merely effortful, a thing to get through. What he hadn't expected was the rest of it. The quality of the light at that hour, still low and golden, before the day got efficient and purposeful. The way the cold air hit his face in a way that felt almost corrective, like a small, necessary jolt back to something real. A dog being walked by a neighbor he'd never spoken to; the brief nod of two people sharing the same unremarkable morning. He didn't think any grand thoughts. But by the time he turned back up his own driveway, something had shifted fractionally in the set of his shoulders. His body was slightly less a stranger.

He kept it small by design. Push-ups after his morning coffee. A plank while his laptop booted. Twenty minutes on his bike before the kids woke up on Saturdays, the neighborhood still dark and unhurried around him. He stopped trying to reclaim his college body — that was someone else's story now — and started building something more honest: a body that worked. That moved without complaint. That didn't betray him when his daughter asked him to play.

Movement stopped being penance for a life lived too sedentarily. It became a practice — a daily return to himself. Not the athlete he used to be, but the man he was actively becoming: present, capable, and alive inside his own skin.

Movement Quiz

Before we get into specifics, take two minutes to answer these questions. Answer honestly so you get a sense of how this past week has actually been for you.

This past week, how satisfied were you with your level of physical activity?

⓪ Very unsatisfied ① Unsatisfied ② Fairly satisfied
③ Very satisfied

How many days did you exercise to the point of sweating or being out of breath?

⓪ Never ① 1–2 days ② 3–4 days ③ Every day

How motivated did you feel about exercising or physical movement?

⓪ Very unmotivated ① Somewhat unmotivated ② Motivated ③ Very motivated

How often did you feel genuinely good because you moved your body?

⓪ Never ① Occasionally ② Often ③ Every day

How many days did you spend time outdoors?

⓪ Never ① 1–2 days ② 3–4 days ③ Every day

Your Score: __________ (Total: 0–15)

- If 0–5: Begin with short, consistent bouts of movement. Frequency before intensity.
- If 6–10: Add variety and address weaker areas — strength, mobility, or cardiovascular capacity.
- If 11–15: Maintain and refine. Focus on quality, longevity, and what you actually enjoy.

What Movement Is

Physical movement is any intentional use of your muscles that increases energy expenditure above what it takes to sit still and contemplate whether to move. It spans the obvious — formal exercise — to the underrated: walking to the store, carrying groceries, gardening, climbing stairs, chasing your dog.

But movement isn't one thing. It's four biological signals, each telling your body something different about how to function:

Cardiovascular capacity

Walking, running, cycling, swimming — is your body's way of training its energy systems for sustained effort. Your entire organism begins to adapt and change. Your heart becomes more efficient. Your body learns to keep going long after the initial discomfort would have stopped an undertrained system.

Strength

Weights, resistance bands, or your own bodyweight — is the signal that tells your muscles and bones they're still expected to be relevant. Without that signal, muscle mass begins to erode in your thirties and accelerates from there. Independence in old age isn't guaranteed. It's earned, incrementally, by asking your body to carry load.

Mobility and flexibility

Stretching, yoga, dynamic movement — quietly determine the range within which your strength can operate. Nobody brags about hip mobility. But its absence is what makes picking something off the floor feel like a negotiation with your own skeleton.

Balance

The most overlooked of the four — is the margin between graceful aging and a fall that changes everything. Train it deliberately, and you stay upright. Neglect it, and gravity eventually collects.

These four categories aren't separate programs. They're an integrated system. The body you build through consistent, varied movement is different in kind — not just degree — from the body that sits still.

And here's the cognitive dimension that most fitness writing misses: movement isn't just good for your body. It's good for the instrument you use to run your life. Regular movement sharpens System 1 for quick, accurate responses while giving System 2 — the planning, decision-making, self-regulating part of your brain — the metabolic fuel it needs to function. Skip movement consistently, and both systems drift toward the path of least resistance. Which, in modern life, usually involves a couch, a screen, and eventually a conversation with a doctor about things that could have been prevented.

Why Movement Is Non-Negotiable

Movement isn't optional background noise. It's the signal that tells every system in your body to stay strong, repair, and adapt. When you move regularly, your heart pumps more efficiently, your muscles and bones receive the message that they're still needed, and your brain receives a continuous supply of oxygen and growth factors that protect its long-term function. When you don't move, your body receives a different message: we're winding down.

The short-term costs are subtle enough to rationalize. Fatigue. Stiffness. A nagging sense that your body is a step behind your intentions. Stairs feel heavier. Energy dips earlier in the day. Mood darkens more frequently. Even one sedentary week measurably dulls cardiovascular stamina and sharpens baseline anxiety.

Over time, the costs compound in ways that become increasingly difficult to reverse. Muscle and bone loss accelerate. Metabolic and cardiovascular risk rise. Balance and coordination fade. What starts as skipped walks becomes an increased probability of falls, fractures, and chronic illness — not as dramatic fate, but as quiet statistical drift in a direction you didn't choose.

The Cost of Neglect

- Persistent fatigue and low stamina: Energy reserves shrink. Even small tasks feel draining by afternoon.
- Stiffness and joint ache: Range of motion contracts. The body starts to feel older than the calendar says.
- Shortness of breath on minimal exertion: Cardiovascular deconditioning happens faster than most people expect — and slower to reverse.
- Declining balance and coordination: Small slips become large risks. The margin for error narrows quietly.
- Everyday tasks becoming effortful: Carrying groceries, standing quickly, climbing stairs — things that should be routine start to feel like challenges.
- Mental strain and emotional fragility: Higher baseline stress, more restless energy, and fewer neurological resources available for resilience.

The Payoff of Consistent Movement

- Greater energy and vitality: Movement is a renewable energy source. The more you do, the more capacity you build to do more.
- Reduced chronic disease risk: Active muscles function like endocrine organs — releasing compounds that regulate

blood sugar, reduce inflammation, and protect cardiovascular health.

- Faster recovery from stress: Exercise trains your nervous system to bounce back more quickly from both physical and emotional strain.

- Confidence in your own body: You trust yourself to carry, climb, sprint, or simply keep up. Independence extends further into old age.

- Cognitive resilience: Regular movement protects memory, attention, and creative capacity well into later decades.

- Emotional steadiness: By regulating dopamine, serotonin, and cortisol, consistent activity lowers the baseline risk of anxiety and depression.

Movement and Long-Term Mental Health

The relationship between movement and mental health runs in both directions — and that bidirectionality is worth being precise about.

When you exercise, your brain releases Brain-Derived Neurotrophic Factor (BDNF), the molecule that keeps neurons flexible, adaptive, and capable of forming new connections. Ratey calls it 'Miracle-Gro for the brain.'[16] Cardiovascular exercise increases blood flow to the prefrontal cortex, the region most responsible for planning, self-regulation, and emotional modulation.[17] Strength training improves executive function.[18] Mind-body practices like yoga and tai chi reduce circulating cortisol and stabilize mood over time.[19]

The vicious loop runs in the other direction too. Inactivity increases baseline cortisol. Elevated cortisol disrupts sleep. Disrupted sleep impairs mood. Impaired mood reduces motivation to move. Reduced movement elevates cortisol. Each turn of the cycle tightens the constraint. What looks like laziness from the outside is often a nervous system that has slowly optimized for stillness because stillness felt safe.

From a systems perspective: inactivity leaves System 1 running anxious and reactive while System 2 becomes sluggish and avoidant. The mental health consequences aren't a side effect of being unfit. They're a direct result of depriving the brain of the chemical environment it was built to receive from a body in motion.

Movement is one of the most evidence-based interventions available for depression, anxiety, and cognitive decline.[20] And unlike most interventions, the side effects are exclusively positive.

Movement Outside - The Compounding Effect

All four types of movement — cardiovascular, strength, mobility, balance — are better when they happen outside. Not marginally. Measurably.

This is not intuition or lifestyle preference. It is what the research consistently shows. Studies comparing equivalent indoor and outdoor exercise find that outdoor movement produces greater reductions in cortisol, larger improvements in mood and self-reported energy, and significantly lower rates of perceived exertion — meaning the same physical work feels easier when it's done outside.[49] Participants who exercise outdoors consistently report higher enjoyment and higher rates of intention to repeat the behavior. The motivational benefit alone matters enormously, because the most effective exercise program is the one you'll actually do again tomorrow.[49]

The mechanisms are specific. Natural light exposure during movement reinforces the circadian signal that governs sleep quality, cortisol timing, and morning alertness the following day. Variable terrain — even the mild unevenness of a sidewalk, a trail, or a park path — engages stabilizing muscles and proprioceptive systems that flat, controlled surfaces cannot. The irregular visual landscape of natural environments engages the brain differently than a gym wall or a treadmill screen: natural patterns occupy and gently stimulate peripheral attention, reducing the ruminative self-referential thinking that indoor movement tends to leave room for. And natural settings, particularly those with trees, water, or open sky, trigger a shift in the autonomic nervous system that compounds the stress-reducing effects of the movement itself. You get the cortisol clearance from exercise, and the cortisol clearance from nature, simultaneously.

There is a specific body of research — pioneered in Japan under the name shinrin-yoku, or forest bathing, and now replicated extensively in Western settings — on what happens when people spend time in wooded or forested environments, even at rest. Blood pressure drops. Cortisol drops. Natural killer cell activity — a marker of immune function — increases for up to a week following a single two-hour walk in trees.[50] The researchers traced part of the mechanism to phytoncides: volatile organic compounds released by trees that humans inhale and that have measurable physiological effects. The forest is not merely a pleasant backdrop. It is, to a nervous system evolved to live in it, a restorative environment with specific biological action.[50]

You do not need to live near a forest. A park with mature trees will produce measurable effects. A route that passes a garden, a green median, or a body of water will produce measurable effects. The research threshold for restoration is lower than most people assume — 20 minutes in a natural setting two to three times per week produces significant and sustained reductions in baseline cortisol.[51] Even brief micro-exposures matter: a 40-second glance at a green rooftop, a few minutes eating lunch outside, the choice of a tree-lined route over a concrete one. Our organism is sensitive. It is waiting for the input.[52]

The practical implication is simple: when you have a choice between moving inside and moving outside, move outside. When you're building new movement habits, build them outside whenever possible — because the lower perceived exertion means you'll start more often, and the higher enjoyment means you'll come back. And when movement isn't on the schedule but a short walk is available, take the walk. The return per minute is among the highest available in this entire book.

How to Build Movement Skills

Knowing that movement matters isn't the same as moving. The science above is necessary context — but information without behavior change is just expensive trivia. What follows is how you build the actual skill.

Movement is practiced, not acquired. You get better at it the same way you get better at anything: through specific goals, deliberate repetition, real feedback, and incremental challenge. Here's how the Four Drivers map onto your actual life.

Start Small

The goal isn't to be impressive. The goal is to be consistent. Small and done beats ambitious and skipped every single time.

- Walk for two minutes after each meal. Your blood sugar will regulate, your gut will thank you, and your nervous system will start associating movement with the already-established habit of eating.

- Five bodyweight squats while the coffee brews. This is not a workout. It is a vote for the identity you're building.

- Master the form of one exercise before turning it into a volume competition. Skill before load. Technique before tonnage.

Shape Your Environment

Willpower runs out. Environment doesn't. The goal is to design your physical space so that the right choice is also the easiest one — and the wrong choice requires deliberate effort to make.

- Workout clothes on the bed. The distance between intention and action should be three steps, not a search through the closet.
- Leave a yoga mat rolled out in your living space. A mat in a drawer gets used occasionally. A mat on the floor gets used.
- Pre-pack your gym bag and place it where you can't avoid seeing it. Out of sight is out of behavior.

Link Habits

You already have behaviors that run on autopilot. The goal is to use them as launch pads. Attach the new behavior to an existing cue and it inherits some of the automaticity that cue already has. System 1 stops arguing. System 2 can stand down.

- 'After I pour my morning coffee, I will do 10 squats.' The coffee is already automatic. The squats catch a ride.
- 'I only listen to [specific podcast or playlist] when I'm moving.' This is temptation bundling — you're not forcing yourself to exercise, you're making exercise the price of admission for something you already want. System 1 does the math and decides movement is worth it.
- Count down out loud — 3, 2, 1 — when it's time to get off the couch. The countdown interrupts the inertia loop before it can complete. It sounds trivial. It works.

Celebrate the Wins

Celebration isn't optional. It's the dopaminergic signal that tells your brain this behavior is worth encoding. The emotional quality of the moment immediately after a behavior determines whether the habit circuit strengthens or stalls. Use it deliberately.

- After any movement — even a short one — pause and acknowledge it. A genuine internal 'good' activates the same reward circuitry as external praise. Your brain doesn't distinguish the source. Use that.

- Keep a movement streak tracker. Visible progress activates the completion drive — the same mechanism that makes you want to finish a nearly-full punch card. Green checkmarks are underrated motivational technology.

- Track skill and form improvements, not just weight lifted or miles covered. Progress isn't always numerical. Getting a push-up cleaner is progress. Recognizing it as progress makes you more likely to practice.

Your Action Steps

1. Start Small

Make the habit feel impossible to fail:

- "On days when I have zero motivation, the one movement I will do no matter what is ____________________ (e.g., walk around the block, do 5 push-ups, stretch for 2 minutes)."

- "I will add movement to my morning by doing ____________________ immediately after ____________________ (e.g., 10 squats after pouring my coffee, a 5-minute walk after breakfast)."

- "This week, I will increase my movement by just __________________ minutes per day — nothing more."
- "My minimum outdoor movement this week, on days when nothing else happens, is __________________ (e.g., a 10-minute walk after lunch, one lap around the block before dinner). It will happen outside, not on a treadmill."

2. Shape Your Environment

Design for the version of yourself who will be tired and unmotivated at 6 p.m.:

- "I will place my __________________ (shoes, yoga mat, resistance band) in __________________ so I see it before I can make an excuse."
- "I will pack my gym bag on __________________ (Sunday night, the night before) and leave it in __________________ (by the door, in my car, on my desk)."
- "I will remove __________________ from my path to movement by __________________ (e.g., lay out workout clothes the night before, move the TV remote away from the couch)."
- *"I will identify one outdoor route I can use within ______ minutes of my home or workplace. I will walk it once this week just to establish it. Familiar routes lower the decision cost of going."*
- *"I will move one outdoor trigger into my sightline: ______________ (e.g., walking shoes near the door, a note on my keys that says 'take the long way')."*

3. Link Habits

Use what already runs on autopilot:

- "Immediately after __________________ (pouring coffee, brushing teeth, sitting down at my desk), I will __________________ (do 10 squats, take a 5-minute walk, stretch my hips for 60 seconds)."

- "I will only listen to __________________ (podcast, playlist, audiobook) when I am moving. This is my temptation bundle."

- "When I feel the urge to sit back down instead of moving, I will count __________________ (5-4-3-2-1) out loud and stand up before I finish."

- "I will pair outdoor movement with __________________ (a call I need to make, a podcast I'm saving, a problem I'm trying to work through). The outdoors is the condition of access, not just the setting."

4. Celebrate the Wins

Reinforce the behavior so your brain encodes it as worth repeating:

- "Immediately after I move — even for 5 minutes — I will say to myself: ____________________________________ (e.g., 'That counts,' 'I showed up for myself today')."

- "I will track my movement by marking __________________ every day I complete my minimum. I will keep this tracker in __________________ (my phone, a wall calendar, a notebook)."

- "If I move for _______ days in a row, I will reward myself with __________________."

My Movement Commitment

Write it down. Specific. Simple. Small enough that you'll actually do it.

New Behavior:
What, specifically, will you do? (Keep it small.)

The Setup:
How will you prepare your environment for success?

The Trigger:
I will do this immediately before/after I:

The Celebration:
I will acknowledge my success by:

Becoming You

At first, movement feels like a chore:

I should exercise more. I should get my steps in. I should finally use that gym membership.

But 'should' rarely survives fatigue, deadlines, or the gravitational pull of the couch. Real strength and vitality don't emerge from occasional heroic workouts. They grow through repeated, ordinary, almost boring acts: taking the stairs instead of the elevator, walking after dinner instead of sitting back down, doing one push-up while the coffee brews.

Each of those acts strengthens not just your muscles but the neural pathways that associate movement with energy rather than effort. Over time, System 2 — the part of you that plans, negotiates, and sets reminders — begins to pass the baton to System 1. Moving stops being a debate. It becomes a default.

You stop seeing yourself as someone trying to exercise. You start seeing yourself as someone who simply moves. Not a former athlete chasing a lost body. A person who has built something more durable: a body that works, that shows up, that doesn't betray you when it counts.

The identity shift is the whole game. You're no longer white-knuckling your way through workouts to burn calories. You're someone whose body and mind expect — and genuinely enjoy — regular movement. Physical activity stops being a reluctant item on your list. It becomes part of who you are: energetic, capable, and alive in your own skin.

Marcus got there. Not with a perfect program. Not all at once. Just one walk around the block, repeated until it became the kind of person he was. So can you.

Nutrition & Hydration

Skill #3: Fuel and Flow

"Every time you eat or drink, you are either feeding disease or fighting it."
— Heather Morgan

Mark

Mark had a running list of shoulds that trailed him like a shadow everywhere he went: I should drink more water. I should stop skipping breakfast. I should cook something that doesn't arrive in a cardboard box with a side of guilt. The list was long and familiar and completely, exhaustingly unactionable.

Most days, the shoulds dissolved before noon. Depression has a particular genius for making the obvious feel impossible — not difficult, not inconvenient, but genuinely, physically impossible in a way that's hard to explain to someone who hasn't felt it. Cooking required decisions he didn't have the bandwidth to make. Water seemed pointless in the abstract way that everything seemed pointless. Takeout was at least predictable, required nothing from him, asked no questions. Food had become purely functional — fuel he barely noticed consuming, often standing over the sink at 10pm, eating cold leftovers directly from the container because sitting down at the table felt, in some way he couldn't fully articulate, like too much effort.

This went on for longer than he told anyone.

Then his therapist suggested something almost insultingly small: pour a glass of water before your morning coffee. Not instead of it. Not a detox. Not a complete overhaul of his relationship with his caffeine. Just — water first, then coffee. He stared at her for a moment, waiting for the rest of the prescription. There wasn't one. That was it.

He did it. It took eleven seconds. The next week, he tried an apple instead of nothing for breakfast. These weren't interventions. They weren't transformations. They were hairline cracks of light in a very thick fog — small enough that depression couldn't marshal a credible argument against them.

The deliberateness of it was exhausting at first. Everything had to be written down, coaxed, manually initiated. But slowly, almost without his permission, a rhythm formed. The water glass lived next to the kettle now — that was just where it lived. Keeping simple food in the house meant meals stopped being emergencies requiring heroic effort. His body, dulled for so long it had nearly gone silent, started sending clearer signals. Thirst. Hunger. Occasionally, something that resembled satisfaction.

Months later, Mark noticed he no longer thought of himself as someone trying to eat better. He was just someone who took care of himself. Depression still showed up — it didn't vanish because he'd started eating apples. But the floor felt sturdier beneath him. He had evidence, sip by sip and meal by meal, that he could meet his own basic needs.

And that quiet competence had begun, slowly, to rewrite the story he told about who he was.

Nutrition & Hydration Quiz

Before we get into specifics, take two minutes to answer these questions. Answer honestly so you get a sense of how this past week has actually been for you.

This past week, how satisfied were you with your nutrition and hydration?

⓪ Very dissatisfied ① Dissatisfied ② Fairly satisfied
③ Very satisfied

How consistent were your eating habits this past week?

⓪ Very inconsistent ① Somewhat inconsistent
② Fairly consistent ③ Very consistent

How many days did you have a deliberate meal plan or intentional food choices?

⓪ No days ① 1–2 days ② 3–4 days ③ Every day

How many days did you eat out of boredom or frustration rather than hunger?

⓪ Every day ① Most days ② A few days ③ No days

How many days did you drink at least six 8-oz glasses of water?

⓪ No days ① 1–2 days ② 3–4 days ③ Every day

Your Score: __________ (Total: 0–15)

- If 0–5: Start with hydration and one whole-food meal per day. Build the floor before you build the house.
- If 6–10: Increase nutritional balance and begin reducing the foods that are working against you.
- If 11–15: Optimize timing and food quality. You have the foundation — now refine it for performance and longevity.

What Nutrition & Hydration Actually Are

Nutrition and hydration are the molecular substrate on which everything else runs. Every neurotransmitter your brain produces, every cell membrane it maintains, every electrical impulse it fires depends on a continuous supply of raw materials: amino acids, fatty acids, glucose, vitamins, minerals, and water. Your body doesn't synthesize these from willpower or good intentions. You either supply them, or you don't. And when you don't, your nervous system begins making compromises — subtle at first, then compounding into something harder to reverse.

There are four categories of nutritional input, each sending different signals to your biology:

Macronutrients

Protein, fats, and carbohydrates — are the structural materials and fuel. Protein provides the amino acids your body uses to rebuild tissue and synthesize neurotransmitters like serotonin and dopamine. Fats form the myelin insulation around every nerve cell and account for roughly 60 percent of your brain's dry weight[21] — a statistic that should make anyone reconsider decades of low-fat advice. Carbohydrates fuel the prefrontal cortex, the seat of System 2 thinking, which burns through glucose faster than any other tissue when you're problem-solving, regulating emotions, or trying not to say the thing you're about to say.

Micronutrients

Vitamins and minerals — are the invisible operators running thousands of enzymatic reactions in the background. B vitamins support energy metabolism and neurotransmitter production. Magnesium regulates the stress response. Zinc and iron affect mood stability and cognitive function. Deficiencies don't announce themselves with alarms. They show up as brain fog, irritability, fatigue, and the vague sense that something is off — symptoms that get attributed to everything except the most likely cause.

Hydration

The most underestimated variable in cognitive performance. Your brain is approximately 73 percent water.[22] Losing just 2 percent of your body's water content — a level of dehydration most people reach before they feel thirsty — measurably impairs attention, working memory, and mood regulation.[23] System 2 becomes sluggish and error-prone. System 1 gets more reactive and impulsive. Chronic under-hydration creates a persistent low-grade cognitive drag that most people attribute to stress, aging, or poor sleep. They're often just thirsty.

Timing and consistency matter more than perfection. Skipping meals creates blood sugar crashes that activate the stress response — cortisol spikes, System 1 reaches for fast energy, and whatever was in front of you nutritionally wins. Regular, balanced eating stabilizes blood glucose and keeps System 2 available when you need executive function most. The goal isn't an optimized meal plan. It's a nervous system that isn't constantly improvising.

Why Nutrition Is the Substrate, Not the Side Note

Nutrition and hydration aren't about calories or macros. They are the chemical preconditions for moment-to-moment functioning. Every hormone your body produces, every neurotransmitter your brain synthesizes, every immune response your system mounts depends on a steady supply of what you eat and drink. Get that supply right and the system runs. Get it consistently wrong and the system compensates in ways that eventually become impossible to ignore.

The Cost of Neglect

- Midday energy crashes: Blood sugar swings spike cortisol and hijack System 1. Every afternoon becomes a negotiation with your own nervous system.

- Brain fog and slow thinking: System 2 runs on glucose. Inconsistent fuel means inconsistent access to the cognitive capacities you need most.

- Mood swings and irritability: Every blood sugar spike is followed by a crash. The emotional fallout is not a character flaw — it's biochemistry.

- Digestive discomfort: Bloating, reflux, and irregularity become constant background noise when the gut microbiome is chronically under-resourced.

- Weakened physical resilience: Skin, hair, muscle tone, and immune function all reflect the quality of the inputs your body is working with.

The Payoff of Consistent Nourishment

- Steady, sustained energy: Without blood sugar rollercoasters, energy stops being a finite resource you ration and becomes something you can rely on.

- Stable mood and emotional regulation: Consistent glucose and adequate neurotransmitter precursors create the neurochemical conditions for emotional steadiness.

- Cognitive sharpness: Memory, focus, and creative capacity all improve when the brain has the raw materials it needs to function at full capacity.

- Better digestion and physical vitality: A well-nourished gut microbiome affects everything from immune function to mood to energy. It's the most underrated organ system in the body.

- Long-term protection: Consistent nutrition and hydration reduce inflammatory load, support hormonal balance, and lower the cumulative risk of cardiovascular disease, metabolic dysfunction, and cognitive decline.

Nutrition, Hydration, and Long-Term Mental Health

The relationship between nutrition and mental health is bidirectional, and the mechanisms are more direct than most people realize.

Your brain produces serotonin, dopamine, and GABA — the neurotransmitters most implicated in mood, motivation, and anxiety regulation — from dietary amino acids. No adequate protein intake, no adequate precursors. Omega-3 fatty acids support the structural integrity of neuronal membranes and regulate inflammatory pathways that are directly linked to depression risk. The gut produces approximately 90 percent of the body's serotonin[24] — meaning the state of your microbiome has a measurable effect on your emotional baseline, independent of what's happening in your brain.

Here's the vicious loop: poor nutrition creates chronic low-grade inflammation. Inflammation is now one of the most robust biological correlates of depression — not as a metaphor, but as a measurable physiological state. Inflammatory cytokines cross the blood-brain barrier and directly impair the synthesis of serotonin and dopamine.[25] Impaired mood reduces motivation and executive function. Reduced executive function makes it harder to shop, cook, or make intentional food choices. Which worsens nutrition. Which sustains the inflammation.

From a systems perspective: nutritional neglect leaves System 1 reactive, impulsive, and metabolically stressed, while System 2 loses the glucose and micronutrient supply it needs to regulate behavior. You end up in a state where the executive capacities required to improve your nutrition are precisely the ones most degraded by poor nutrition. It's a trap with a biological mechanism. Recognizing the mechanism is the first step out of it.

Food and water (nourishment) isn't optional. It's the substrate that makes everything else — including the willingness to try — chemically possible.

How to Build Nutrition & Hydration Skills

Knowing that nutrition matters isn't the same as eating well. The science above is the map — but maps don't move you. What follows is the practice.

Eating well is a skill, not a character trait. You get better at it the same way you get better at anything: through specific goals, deliberate repetition, real feedback, and incremental challenge. Here's how the Four Drivers translate into your actual kitchen, your actual schedule, and your actual energy level at 7 p.m.

Start Small

For this chapter more than any other, small means genuinely small. When System 2 is depleted — by depression, stress, or just a hard week — the bar for what's executable drops dramatically. Design for the hardest version of your day, not the easiest.

- Swap one salty/cheesy snack for a piece of fruit and a handful of nuts. Not every snack. One. Your microbiome will register the signal even if you don't.

- Add one extra glass of water at the same time every morning. Consistency matters more than volume. Hydration is a habit before it's a quantity.

- Add one vegetable to dinner. Not a vegetable overhaul. One. Pick whichever one requires the least effort to prepare and put it on the plate.

Shape Your Environment

Most food decisions aren't decisions — they're defaults. Whatever is visible, accessible, and requires the least effort is what gets eaten. Design your food environment around that reality instead of fighting it.

- Keep a full water bottle on your desk or counter. You don't need to remember to hydrate if the water is already in front of you. Out of sight is out of intake.

- Pre-cut vegetables and store them at eye level in the fridge. Impulse eating isn't the enemy — it's the opportunity. Make the impulse reach for something that works.

- Move the healthiest options to the front of the pantry and the fridge. Put the harder choices behind them. You're not restricting — you're reordering the default.

Link Habits

You already have dozens of behaviors that run on autopilot every day. Each one is a potential anchor point for a nutritional habit. The goal isn't to build a new routine from scratch — it's to attach a new behavior to something that already fires reliably.

- Pair your morning coffee with a full glass of water first. Caffeine without hydration accelerates dehydration. The coffee is already automatic — let the water catch a ride on that habit.

- After every bathroom break, drink a small glass of water. Yes, this creates a self-reinforcing loop. That's the point. Frequency of the cue determines the strength of the habit.

- Every time you pack lunch or prep dinner, add one fiber-rich food — beans, lentils, dark leafy greens. Not as a rule to follow, but as a default to install.

Celebrate the Wins

For someone navigating depression or chronic stress, self-acknowledgment can feel hollow or performative. It's neither. The brief moment of recognition immediately after a positive behavior fires a dopaminergic signal that strengthens the habit circuit at the neurological level. This isn't motivation. It's biology. Use it.

- Eat the same, healthy meal once a week. Notice what consistent nutrition feels like.

- Log your water intake in an app for one week — then delete the app and keep the habit. The log trains the awareness. The awareness becomes the habit.

- Notice when you've gone a whole day without a sugar crash. That's blood sugar stability — which is a measurable physiological achievement. Name it as such. System 1 responds to acknowledgment even when System 2 is skeptical.

- Keep a short running list of meals that make you feel good two hours later, not just in the moment. Over time, this list becomes your personal evidence base for what nourishment actually looks like for your body specifically.

Your Action Steps

1. Start Small

Make the first change so small it would be embarrassing to skip:

- "The one nutritional change I will make this week, no matter what, is ________________ (e.g., drink one glass of water when I wake up, add one piece of fruit to my morning, eat lunch sitting down instead of standing)."
- "Instead of trying to overhaul my diet, I will focus only on ________________ this week (e.g., breakfast, afternoon snacking, hydration)."
- "On days when I have no energy to cook, my minimum viable meal is ________________ (e.g., yogurt and fruit, eggs and toast, a handful of nuts and an apple). I will always have these ingredients available."

2. Shape Your Environment

Design your kitchen and workspace for the version of yourself who is tired and depleted at 6 p.m.:

- "I will place ________________ (water bottle, fruit bowl, pre-cut vegetables) in ________________ (on my desk, on the kitchen counter, at eye level in the fridge) so it's the first thing I reach for."
- "I will move ________________ (chips, candy, processed snacks) to ________________ (a high shelf, a closed cabinet, out of the house) so accessing them requires deliberate effort."
- "I will prep ________________ (hard-boiled eggs, cut vegetables, portioned nuts) on ________________

(Sunday evening, Monday morning) so healthy options are ready when I don't want to think."

3. Link Habits

Attach new nutritional behaviors to routines that already run automatically:

- "Immediately after ___________________ (pouring my morning coffee, sitting down at my desk, finishing my morning workout), I will ___________________ (drink a glass of water, eat a piece of fruit, take my vitamins)."
- "Every time I ___________________ (go to the bathroom, finish a meeting, take a work break), I will ___________________ (drink a small glass of water, eat a small snack if it's been more than 3 hours, refill my water bottle)."
- "When I prep dinner, I will automatically add ___________________ (one vegetable, one fiber source, one protein) to whatever I'm already making — no separate meal planning required."

4. Celebrate the Wins

Reinforce the behaviors your brain needs to encode as worth repeating:

- "When I choose a nourishing option over a depleting one, I will take five seconds to say to myself: ___________________ (e.g., 'That's what taking care of myself looks like,' 'That counts')."
- "I will track my ___________________ (water intake, vegetable servings, consistent meals) for one week using ___________________ (an app, a tally on a sticky note, a

habit tracker) to build awareness before I make it automatic."

- "If I maintain my minimum nutrition habit for _______ days in a row, I will reward myself with __________________."

My Nutrition & Hydration Commitment

Write it down. Specific. Simple. Small enough that you'll actually do it.

New Behavior:
What, specifically, will you do? (Keep it genuinely small.)

The Setup:
How will you prepare your environment for success?

The Trigger:
I will do this immediately before/after I:

The Celebration:
I will acknowledge my success by:

Becoming You

At first, eating well feels like a list of failures:

I should cook more. I should drink more water. I should stop skipping breakfast.

'Should' doesn't stand a chance against late nights, empty fridges, and a brain that's running low on executive resources. Real nourishment isn't built on guilt or grand declarations. It's built one sip, one meal, one unremarkable choice at a time. A glass of water before coffee. A lunch that doesn't come in a crinkly bag. A piece of fruit instead of nothing. Each act sends a signal to your nervous system: we have what we need. We're not in crisis. We can function.

At first, System 2 does all the work — the reminders, the shopping lists, the moment-by-moment decisions. It feels effortful and deliberate and sometimes inconvenient. But the repetitions accumulate. Each choice lays down a thin layer of neural infrastructure. Until one day, reaching for the water bottle is just what you do. Until assembling a simple meal feels less like a task and more like a reflex.

System 2 passes the baton to System 1. And what once required willpower becomes just... you.

You're no longer someone trying to eat better or working on drinking enough water. You're simply the kind of person who fuels their body with some degree of care and intention. The floor feels sturdier. The fog lifts a little more often. And that steadiness — earned through the most ordinary of habits — is not a destination. It's who you've become.

Mark got there. Not through a meal plan or a nutrition overhaul. Through a glass of water before his morning coffee, repeated until it became the kind of person he was. So can you.

Self-Care

Skill #4: The Art of Inner Leadership

"Mastering others is strength. Mastering yourself is true power."
— Lao Tzu

Arthur

Arthur was 48 and felt like his life ran on autopilot — but not the smooth, cruising kind. More like a malfunctioning autopilot that banked hard into turbulence every time stress appeared. He snapped at his kids over minor messes — a backpack left in the hallway, a glass left on the wrong counter — and felt the guilt of it settle into his chest before the words had even finished leaving his mouth. He stayed up late doomscrolling even though he knew, with the weary certainty of long experience, exactly how it would make him feel the next morning. He woke up most days already behind, already braced, as if sleep were something that happened to him rather than something he chose.

Self-care, to Arthur, was a phrase that belonged to other people. People in yoga pants. People without mortgages and quarterly reviews and kids who needed rides at inconvenient times.

He told himself the usual things — *I should be more patient, I should stop checking email in bed, I should eat something that isn't assembled in forty seconds* — but should is a fragile creature. It rarely survives a long day at work followed by traffic and the stack of bills on the kitchen counter that he'd been moving from one side to the other for three weeks without opening.

One night, while brushing his teeth, Arthur decided to try something almost embarrassingly small. When he felt the urge to check his phone in bed, he would first take one slow breath. Just one. No app required. Just one breath. Simply because it felt kind.

The first night, he took that breath and grabbed the phone anyway. The second night, he took that breath and set the phone down for five minutes before picking it up. By the end of the week, the pause had stretched long enough that he fell asleep with the screen dark and untouched on the nightstand.

No epiphany. No dramatic turning point. Just small, almost invisible cracks forming in the armor of old habit. The breath before the snapped reply. The pause before the sarcastic comment he would have regretted. The choice, three nights a week, to take a walk after dinner instead of liquefying into the couch.

He wouldn't have called those walks a practice. They were just the thing he did instead of the thing that was making him worse. But he noticed — and this surprised him — that the walk itself had a specific quality that sitting in the house didn't. The simple fact of being outside, with air that moved and light that changed depending on the cloud cover, produced something he couldn't quite name. Less like feeling better. More like the noise had been turned down slightly. His thoughts stopped chasing each other in circles and started going somewhere, if only around the block. By the time he got back, whatever had been vibrating in his chest had quieted enough that he could make a different choice about the rest of the evening.

Over months, something shifted in a way that was hard to name until it was already done. What had required reminders and gritted teeth began to feel ordinary. The pause before the email reply wasn't a discipline anymore — it was just what he did. A weekend nap stopped requiring justification. Reading in the evening became the default, replacing the scrolling that had left him wired and vaguely ashamed.

Arthur wasn't chasing shoulds anymore. He had become someone who tended to his own reserves the way he'd learned to tend to everything else that mattered — steadily, without drama, before the warning light came on.

For the first time in years, he wasn't just surviving his days.

He was steering them.

Self-Care Quiz

Before we get into specifics, take two minutes to answer these questions. Answer honestly so you get a sense of how this past week has actually been for you.

This past week, how satisfied were you with your self-care habits?

⓪ Very dissatisfied ① Dissatisfied ② Fairly satisfied
③ Very satisfied

How often did you engage in non-work activities — reading, music, hobbies, rest?

⓪ No days ① 1–2 days ② 3–4 days ③ Every day

How often did you check work email or do work-related tasks within 1–2 hours of bedtime?

⓪ Every night ① Most nights ② A few nights ③ Not at all

How many days did you engage in basic personal hygiene — showering, brushing teeth, clean clothes?

⓪ No days ① 1–2 days ② 3–4 days ③ Every day

How often did you practice personal reflection — meditation, journaling, breathwork, or quiet time?

⓪ No days ① 1–2 days ② 3–4 days ③ Every day

Your Score:__________ (Total: 0–15)

- If 0–5: Start with awareness — one daily self-check-in to notice your internal state before reacting to it.
- If 6–10: Strengthen your regulation tools. Identify your two or three most reliable ways to come back to baseline.
- If 11–15: Maintain through intentional practice. The goal now is depth and consistency, not acquisition of new tools.

What Self-Care Actually Is

Self-care isn't indulgence. It isn't a spa day or a productivity hack or the thing you do when you've finally earned enough rest. It's the ongoing practice of tending to the internal conditions that allow you to function, feel, and heal — the daily maintenance of the system you live inside.

From a biological standpoint, self-care is the practice of intentionally cultivating what researchers call the 'window of tolerance' — the range of nervous system activation within which your brain can function at its best.[26] Inside that window, System 2 is available: you can think clearly, regulate emotion, make decisions that align with your values. Outside it, System 1 takes over — and System 1 is optimized for outrunning predators, not for navigating difficult conversations, work deadlines, or a grocery store at 5 p.m. on a Friday.

When the window narrows — under stress, exhaustion, emotional overload, or unmet basic needs — System 1 hijacks the controls. You snap. You scroll. You reach for whatever provides the fastest relief, regardless of the cost. Not because you lack discipline or character. Because your nervous system is doing exactly what it was designed to do when it perceives threat. Self-care is how you widen the window so that survival mode isn't your default operating system.

Self-care rests on three trainable capacities:

- **Awareness** — noticing your internal state with the curiosity of a researcher rather than the judgment of a critic. What's actually happening right now, in your body and mind, before you react?

- **Regulation** — supporting your nervous system toward baseline rather than muscling through overwhelm or numbing it into silence. This is the breath, the walk, the pause. The small acts of physiological reset.

- **Alignment** — choosing, again and again, the behaviors that serve your long-term well-being rather than defaulting to whatever short-term relief System 1 is offering.

None of these are fixed traits. All three are skills that get sharper with practice. Self-care isn't a switch you flip. It's a garden you tend — and the garden becomes more habitable the more consistently you show up for it.

One of the most underappreciated — and most accessible — tools for nervous system regulation has been available for the entirety of human existence, requires no equipment, and costs nothing: contact with the natural world.

When you walk through a park, or sit near water, or watch light move through leaves, your brain isn't working hard to pay attention. It's drawn in gently, without cost. This distinction matters because directed attention — the kind you use to write emails, manage schedules, make decisions, and navigate difficult conversations — depletes. It runs down like a battery. And unlike a battery, it can't simply be recharged by stopping. It needs specific inputs to restore. Natural environments are one of those inputs. They engage a different attentional mode entirely, allowing the depleted voluntary system to recover while the involuntary system is quietly, pleasurably occupied.[53]

For the window of tolerance, this is directly relevant. The restorative effect of natural environments isn't just about mental fatigue — it produces measurable reductions in cortisol, lowers heart rate, and shifts the autonomic nervous system from sympathetic (alert, mobilized, vigilant) toward parasympathetic (restored, regulated, safe). These are the same physiological markers that indicate a widening window of tolerance. A walk outside, in other words, is not a distraction from your self-care practice. In many cases, it is your self-care practice.[44]

Why Self-Care Is the Foundation, Not the Reward

Self-care is not the soft alternative to discipline. It is the foundation that makes discipline biologically possible.

When your nervous system is dysregulated — when you're running on too little sleep, too much cortisol, and not enough of anything that replenishes you — System 1 doesn't just influence your behavior. It runs it. The prefrontal cortex goes offline under chronic stress in ways that are measurable and well-documented.[27] Executive function degrades. Impulse control weakens. The capacity to tolerate discomfort, delay gratification, or choose the harder right thing over the easier wrong one all depend on a nervous system that isn't already in survival mode.

The Cost of Neglect

- Impulsive decisions: You act before your prefrontal cortex has a chance to weigh in — and live with the consequences after.
- Narrowed tolerance: Small stressors trigger disproportionate reactions because the window of tolerance is already nearly closed.
- Chronic procrastination: System 1 wins the argument for short-term comfort, every time, because System 2 doesn't have the fuel to counter it.
- Fragile habits: Long-term goals get consistently sabotaged by momentary urges because the regulatory capacity to hold the tension is depleted.
- Emotional volatility: Relationships bear the cost of a nervous system running reactions instead of responses.

The Payoff of Consistent Self-Care

- Steadier emotional baseline: Stress triggers don't immediately hijack your behavior. You have a moment — and in that moment, you have a choice.

- Aligned daily choices: What you do each day increasingly reflects what you actually value, rather than what System 1 reached for under pressure.

- Greater resilience under stress: A wider window of tolerance means you can stay functional in conditions that previously would have shut you down.

- Cascading improvements across other non-negotiables: Sleep, nutrition, movement, and relationships all improve when self-regulation capacity increases. Self-care is the multiplier.

- Identity consolidation: You become, over time, the kind of person who is trusted, consistent, and steady — by others, and by yourself.

Self-Care and Long-Term Mental Health

The relationship between self-care and mental health is bidirectional — and the direction it runs depends almost entirely on which side of the window you're on.

When self-care is consistent, the window stays open. The nervous system has enough resources to process difficult emotions rather than being overwhelmed by them. The prefrontal cortex can stay online long enough to interrupt automatic patterns, choose different responses, and build the kind of reflective capacity that makes therapy, medication, and behavioral change actually work. Self-care doesn't replace treatment. It creates the neurological conditions under which treatment can take hold.

Here is the vicious loop that neglected self-care creates: dysregulation narrows the window. A narrowed window makes impulsive, avoidant, or self-destructive behavior more likely. Those behaviors — the late-night scrolling, the skipped meals, the isolation, the reactive outbursts — increase shame and cortisol load. Increased shame and cortisol further dysregulate the nervous system. The window narrows further. The loop tightens.

For people with PTSD, this loop is particularly vicious. Trauma already narrows the window dramatically — the nervous system is primed for threat, hypervigilant, and quick to move into fight, flight, or freeze. Neglecting self-care in this context doesn't just maintain the problem. It actively reinforces the neural pathways of dysregulation, making them more automatic and harder to interrupt over time.

Self-care is the practice of keeping the window open — or, when it has narrowed, of widening it again. Not through force. But rather, through the accumulated weight of small, consistent acts of tending. One breath. One walk. One night without the phone. Over time, the window widens. When the window widens, everything else becomes possible.

How to Build Self-Care Skills

Self-care is harder to operationalize than sleep or movement because its primary domain is internal. You can't simply schedule awareness. You can't put regulation on a timer. What you can do is build the external conditions — the environment, the triggers, the small wins — that make the internal practice more likely to happen. That's what the Four Drivers do here.

These aren't hacks for becoming a calmer person. They're the scaffolding that holds up the practice while the practice is still fragile. Use them until you don't need them anymore — which is when you'll realize the practice has become you.

Start Small

The goal of starting small in self-care is not to build gradually toward something larger. The goal is to create a first rep so low-stakes that your nervous system doesn't treat it as a threat. One breath. One pause. One ten-second delay. The circuit doesn't care how small the rep is. It just needs the rep.

- Spend two minutes on your most challenging task before anything else each morning. Not to complete it — just to make contact with it. Momentum starts with contact, not completion.
- Choose one self-regulation act per day — a pause before a reply, a breath before a reaction, a brief check-in with your body before you move to the next thing. One. Not a practice. A single rep.
- When you feel a strong impulse — to scroll, to snack, to avoid — delay acting on it by ten seconds. Just ten. The space between stimulus and response is where self-mastery lives. You're practicing inhabiting that space.

Shape Your Environment

When your window is narrow and System 2 is running low, your environment makes most of your decisions for you. Design it so those decisions point toward regulation rather than away from it.

- Keep a visible reminder of your current intention or value in your workspace — a word, a phrase, a question. Not as inspiration, but as an orientation cue. What you see regularly, you act toward.
- Place a cue card with your top daily priority where you'll encounter it first thing in the morning, before the day has had a chance to take over.

- Remove the primary source of your most common self-regulation failure from your immediate environment during your highest-risk hours. Phone in another room. App deleted. Temptation physically out of reach. You're not testing your willpower — you're not wasting it on a fight you don't need to have.

- "I will identify one outdoor space — a park bench, a route around the block, a spot in a garden — that I can reach within _______ minutes of my home or workplace. When I feel my window narrowing — when I notice the impulsive reach for the phone, the sharpness before a reply, the flatness settling in — this is the space I will go to for _______ minutes before I act. I am not escaping the problem. I am restoring the capacity to handle it."

Link Habits

Self-regulation practices are most fragile as standalone behaviors — they're easy to forget, easy to deprioritize, easy to skip when the day is already demanding. Attach them to something that already runs automatically and they inherit the momentum of that existing habit.

- After you make your morning coffee — before you check your phone, before you open your email — review your top three priorities for the day. Thirty seconds. The coffee is already automatic. Let the review catch a ride.

- Pair a self-control practice — avoiding a specific trigger, taking a brief pause, doing one thing you've been avoiding — with a small, genuinely enjoyable follow-up activity. You're not bribing yourself. You're training your brain to associate the hard thing with a reward that follows it.

- Use the 5-4-3-2-1 countdown to initiate a difficult or uncomfortable task before System 1 generates a sufficient reason not to. Count down out loud. Move before you finish. Interrupt the avoidance loop before it completes.

Celebrate the Wins

Self-care victories are mostly invisible. Nobody claps when you take the breath instead of sending the reactive email. Nobody notices when you put the phone down. The internal acknowledgment is therefore doing all of the reinforcement work — and it needs to be deliberate, because it won't happen automatically. Use it. It's your most powerful tool.

- Acknowledge every act of self-regulation, no matter how small. The pause before the reply. The breath before the reaction. Each one is a rep. Each rep is a vote for the identity you're building. Name it as such.

- Keep a running log of intentional actions — not as a productivity metric but as evidence. When you doubt that you're making progress, the log is your counter-argument.

- Treat each successful self-regulation rep as skill-building rather than willpower — because that's what it is. You're not testing your character. You're training your nervous system. The difference in framing changes what failure means: a rep missed is just a missed rep, not a verdict.

Your Action Steps

1. Start Small

Choose one rep so small your nervous system won't treat it as a threat:

- "The one self-regulation practice I will do every day this week, no matter what, is ____________________ (e.g., take one slow breath before checking my phone, pause for five seconds before sending any reactive message, spend two minutes on my hardest task before opening email)."

- "When I feel the urge to ___________________ (scroll, snack, avoid, snap), I will wait _______ seconds before acting on it. Just _______ seconds."

- "The smallest possible version of my self-care practice — the one I can do even on my worst day — is ___________________."

2. Shape Your Environment

Design your environment to do the regulation work your willpower can't always sustain:

- "I will place ___________________ (a word, a phrase, a question, a photo) in ___________________ (my workspace, my bathroom mirror, my phone lock screen) as a daily orientation cue."

- "During my highest-risk hours for ___________________ (scrolling, reactive messaging, avoidance), I will remove ___________________ from my immediate environment by ___________________."

- "I will set up my morning environment so that the first thing I encounter each day is ___________________ rather than ___________________ (e.g., my journal rather than my phone, my priorities list rather than my inbox)."

3. Link Habits

Attach your self-care practice to something that already runs automatically:

- "Immediately after ___________________ (making my coffee, sitting down at my desk, finishing lunch), I will

____________________ (review my top three priorities, take three slow breaths, write one sentence in my journal)."

- "I will pair ____________________ (my most avoided task, my most challenging self-regulation practice) with ____________________ (a small enjoyable activity that follows it) so my brain learns to associate the hard thing with something good."
- "When I notice the urge to ____________________ (avoid, react, numb), I will count ____________________ out loud and then ____________________ before I act on the urge."

4. Celebrate the Wins

Give your nervous system the signal that self-regulation is safe, possible, and worth repeating:

- "Every time I successfully pause before reacting, I will take five seconds to say to myself: ____________________ (e.g., 'I have a choice here,' 'That's a rep,' 'I'm building this')."
- "I will keep a log of ____________________ (intentional pauses, completed difficult tasks, self-regulation wins) in ____________________ (a notebook, my phone, a habit tracker) so my progress is visible rather than abstract."
- "If I maintain my self-care practice for ________ days in a row, I will reward myself with ____________________."

My Self-Care Commitment

Write it down. Specific. Simple. Small enough that it's hard to talk yourself out of before you've done it.

New Behavior:
What, specifically, will you do? In what situation?

The Setup:
How will you prepare your environment to support this practice?

The Trigger:
I will do this immediately before/after I:

The Celebration:
I will acknowledge my success by:

Becoming You

At first, self-care feels like an aspiration:

I want to feel calmer before I respond. I want more focus. I want to stop numbing out at night.

But aspiration collapses under the speed of stress. System 1 moves faster than any intention. Real self-care isn't built through resolve — it's built through tiny, repeated acts of tending. A single breath to settle the body before speaking. A moment to write down what's crowding the mind so it doesn't have to hold it anymore. The choice to take a walk rather than collapse into the couch — not forever, just tonight, just this once.

Each act is small. Imperfect. Human. But each one is a rep. And each rep is a message to your nervous system: we can do this. We don't have to react. We have a choice here.

Slowly, the reps accumulate. The breath becomes a reflex. The pause feels less foreign. The urge to self-soothe in ways that cost you loses some of its grip. System 2 — the deliberate part of you that chose the breath, set the phone down, took the walk — begins to pass the baton to System 1. What once required effort becomes texture. What once felt like discipline begins to feel like home.

You are no longer someone overwhelmed by every impulse and stressor, white-knuckling your way through the day. You are someone who tends to themselves. Someone who cares for the system they live inside. Self-care stops being a fix you reach for when things fall apart. It becomes the homebase you return to, again and again, because it's where you actually live.

Arthur got there. Not through an epiphany. Through one breath taken before he reached for his phone, repeated until it became the kind of man he was. So can you.

Physical Environment

Skill #5: The Spaces That Shape You

"Your environment will eat your goals and plans for breakfast."
— Peter Drucker

Daniel

For years, Daniel told himself he could think past the clutter. The stack of unopened mail on the kitchen counter that had been there so long it had become part of the landscape. The laundry in semi-permanent piles on the bedroom chair — that chair, the one in every apartment, that exists solely to accumulate things that don't have anywhere else to go. The desk buried under charging cords and old receipts and papers he kept meaning to file. None of it was that bad, he told himself. He was a smart guy. Surely his brain could power through a messy backdrop.

It couldn't. It was just doing it quietly, invisibly, in the background — spending processing power he didn't know he was spending.

One morning, running late, he tripped over the same pair of shoes he'd been stepping around for a week. Something about the third time made it different. He bent down, moved them to the rack by the door — a rack that existed for exactly this purpose — and, while he was at it, cleared a small corner of the entryway. Moved the shoes, stacked the bags, hung up the coat that had been draped over the banister since Tuesday. Two minutes, maybe three.

The relief was absurdly disproportionate to the effort. That was what stopped him. Not the tidiness — the feeling. Like a sound he'd stopped hearing had finally gone silent.

The next morning he opened the blinds as soon as he got up, something he hadn't done in months. Light came through in long strips across the floor and he stood in it for a moment before making coffee. He stayed longer than he'd intended to — not doing anything, just standing where the light was, watching it move slowly across the floor until the coffee finished brewing. It was the first time in months he had stood still in his own home without reaching for something.

A few days later, he bought a single small plant for his desk — something green and alive in a space that had felt neither. Small moves, deliberate at first, almost embarrassingly modest. But each one shifted something in the air around him. It softened the low-frequency noise his nervous system had been running in the background without his permission. Returned a sliver of quiet he hadn't realized he'd been missing until it came back.

Over weeks, the deliberate effort dissolved into habit. He no longer needed to remind himself to clear the counter before bed or reset his desk at the end of the day. It became simply how he lived — unremarkable, automatic, his way.

Daniel stopped thinking of himself as someone who should get more organized. He had become a man whose environment worked with him instead of silently grinding against him.

And the shift reached further than his apartment. With less ambient stress eating at the edges of his attention, he found himself more patient at work, more present in conversations, more at ease inside his own head. Clearing his surroundings hadn't solved everything — the hard things remained hard. But it had removed a thousand tiny pebbles from his shoes.

He could finally walk forward without the weight of them.

Physical Environment Quiz

Before we get into specifics, take two minutes to answer these questions. Answer honestly so you get a sense of how this past week has actually been for you.

This past week, how satisfied were you with your physical surroundings?

⓪ Very dissatisfied ① Dissatisfied ② Fairly satisfied ③ Very satisfied

How safe did you feel in your daily physical spaces this past week?

⓪ Not at all safe ① Somewhat safe ② Fairly safe ③ Very safe

How conducive was your physical environment to feeling like your best self?

⓪ Not at all ① Somewhat ② Fairly ③ Very much so

How often did you clean, straighten, or organize your home?

⓪ Never ① 1–2 days ② 3–4 days ③ Every day

How well did your physical surroundings match your values and aesthetic?

⓪ Not at all ① Somewhat ② Fairly well ③ Very well

Your Score: __________ (Total: 0–15)

- If 0–5: Start with one space that matters most to your daily function. Clear it, then stop. One space, done well, is enough to begin.
- If 6–10: Optimize for both form and function. Address the spaces that create the most friction in your daily routine.
- If 11–15: Maintain and fine-tune for evolving needs. Environments drift without attention. Regular small resets prevent large interventions.

What Your Physical Environment Actually Does

Your Physical Environment is the sum of the spaces you inhabit most — your home, your workspace, your car, the corner of the café where you always sit. It is not background scenery. It is the operating system on which your nervous system runs. And like any operating system, it can either facilitate smooth processing or quietly crash processes in the background without ever triggering an error message you can see.

Your brain is a voracious and indiscriminate data collector. System 1 scans every environment continuously — absorbing light levels, temperature, sound, smell, color, and above all the degree of order or disorder — and feeds that information directly into your stress response, energy levels, and mood. This is not a conscious process. A cluttered desk doesn't register as a problem you're aware of. It registers as a low-level threat signal in the neural basement — a blinking warning light that never turns off, drawing a small but continuous allocation of cognitive resources away from whatever you're actually trying to do.

System 2, meanwhile, believes it's running the show. It isn't. It's heavily influenced by whatever System 1 has been marinating in all day. If your environment is disorganized, dim, or noisy, your deliberate reflective mind is already operating at a deficit before you've made a single conscious choice. It's not that you lack willpower or focus. It's that you're trying to do precise work with an instrument that's already been degraded by its surroundings.

A well-designed environment doesn't happen by accident. It's the result of deliberate choices about what to include, what to remove, and how to arrange what remains. The operating principle is simple: reduce friction for the behaviors you want, increase friction for the ones you don't. Place the running shoes by the door. Put the phone charger in another room. Let the architecture do the work that willpower can't sustain.

Every object, sound, and sight in your space either adds value or taxes your attention. In a world already saturated with stimuli, your environment can function as an ally — a physical arrangement that keeps your priorities visible and your distractions distant — or as one more competing voice pulling you toward whatever is most immediately present. The difference is whether you shape your environment, or your environment shapes you.

The Natural Environment You Already Have Access To

Most environmental design thinking — including most of what you'll find in this chapter — focuses on the interior: the surfaces, the light, the arrangement of objects, the reduction of clutter. All of that matters. But it addresses only the built environment, and the built environment is where humans have spent the vast majority of their time for the past several thousand years. Our nervous systems were built in a much older environment, one that the research on restorative environments keeps pointing us back to: the natural world.

The psychologists Roger Ulrich and Rachel Kaplan have independently established what has become one of the more durable findings in environmental psychology: exposure to natural settings — trees, water, open sky, plants, soil — produces reliable and measurable reductions in physiological stress markers. Cortisol drops. Heart rate lowers. Blood pressure falls. The nervous system shifts toward the parasympathetic recovery state. These effects occur at low doses and without effort. You don't need to try to relax in a natural environment. The environment does the work.

Ulrich's landmark 1984 study — comparing surgical recovery times for hospital patients whose windows faced a brick wall versus a small stand of trees — found that the tree-view patients recovered faster, required less pain medication, and had fewer post-surgical complications.[54] A window. Trees. Measurable clinical outcomes. The natural environment isn't a wellness preference. For a nervous system calibrated in it, it's a functional input with specific physiological action.

For the interior environment, this translates practically. Natural light is the most powerful environmental input available for mood, circadian regulation, and cognitive performance — more so than any bulb or fixture. Living plants in a space have documented effects on air quality, attention, and the perception of stress.[55] Views of natural elements — even a small garden, even a sky visible through a window — reduce baseline cortisol compared to views of built structures alone.[44] Sounds of natural environments — water, birdsong, wind — have measurably different effects on the autonomic nervous system than urban noise.

You cannot always control whether you have a park outside your door. You can almost always control whether you open the blinds.

Why Environment Is the Invisible Architecture of Behavior

Your physical environment is not the backdrop to your life. It is one of its primary determinants. Every light, smell, sound, and object in your space sends a continuous stream of cues to your nervous system — cues that influence your stress levels, your attention, your mood, and the behaviors your brain defaults to when System 2 isn't actively overriding them.

System 1 reads clutter as an unresolved threat. It reads dim light as reduced capacity. It reads noise as demand. None of these readings are conscious — they happen below the threshold of awareness, in the same subcortical circuits that once scanned the savanna for movement in the grass. System 2, running on the degraded fuel that System 1's continuous background stress leaves behind, has less capacity for the deliberate, reflective work that planning, focus, and self-regulation require. Both systems sputter when the environment fights them.

The Cost of Neglect

- Cognitive drag: Clutter and disorder create a continuous low-level attentional tax — paid whether or not you notice the clutter consciously.
- Decision fatigue: Disorganized environments multiply micro-decisions throughout the day, depleting System 2 before it reaches the decisions that actually matter.
- Chronic background stress: Every unresolved pile, every dim corner, every obstacle is a small cortisol stimulus. Multiply by eight hours and the load compounds.
- Degraded habits: The environment that pulls against your intentions wins more often than your intentions do. You cannot out-willpower a bad environment indefinitely.
- Reduced creativity: Cognitive bandwidth spent scanning for order is bandwidth not available for the generative work that requires a quiet, clear mind.

The Payoff of a Supportive Environment

- Cognitive clarity: A clear, ordered space reduces attentional residue and makes the kind of focused work that matters feel easier and more sustainable.
- Behavioral momentum: When your environment is aligned with your intentions, desired behaviors become the default rather than the achievement.
- Lower baseline stress: A calm, organized, well-lit space measurably reduces cortisol and widens the window of

tolerance — the same mechanism discussed in the Self-Care chapter.

- More energy: Natural light, good air quality, and ergonomic design are not luxuries — they are inputs that directly affect physical and cognitive performance.
- Resilient routines: Environments that support your habits make those habits more durable under stress — the architecture holds even when your motivation doesn't.

Environment and Long-Term Mental Health

The relationship between physical environment and mental health operates through mechanisms that are more concrete and more powerful than most people realize — and more relevant to clinical populations than the wellness literature typically acknowledges.

The most direct mechanism is cortisol load. Environmental stressors — noise, clutter, poor lighting, temperature extremes, crowding — activate the hypothalamic-pituitary-adrenal axis and produce measurable increases in cortisol.[28] A single stressor produces a single cortisol pulse. A day spent in a chronically disorganized, noisy, or unsafe environment produces a sustained elevation in baseline cortisol that compounds across weeks and months into what researchers call allostatic load: the cumulative biological wear from chronic stress exposure. Allostatic load is associated with increased risk of depression, anxiety, cardiovascular disease, and accelerated cognitive aging.[29]

For people with depression, the environment-mood relationship runs in both directions. Depression reduces the motivation to maintain physical order; physical disorder increases the background stress that worsens depression. The pile of laundry that never gets done is simultaneously a symptom and a cause — each day it remains, it adds a small increment of unresolved demand to an already depleted system. This is not a moral failing. It is a feedback loop with a physical address.

For people with PTSD, the physical environment carries particular clinical weight. The threat-detection system is already running at elevated sensitivity — the nervous system is primed to read ambiguous signals as dangerous. An environment that is physically chaotic, unsafe, or unpredictable adds signal to an already over-activated system. Conversely, research on restorative environments — spaces characterized by order, natural elements, low stimulation, and felt safety — consistently shows reductions in physiological stress markers and improvements in mood and cognitive function.[30] For trauma survivors, a safe and ordered physical space is not a comfort. It is a clinical intervention.

Here is the vicious loop: environmental disorder increases cortisol and attentional drain. Elevated cortisol reduces motivation and executive function. Reduced executive function makes it harder to address the disorder. The disorder remains and intensifies. The loop tightens. One cleared surface — two minutes of effort — introduces a counter-force. Not enough to break the loop immediately. Enough to demonstrate that it can be broken. And that demonstration is its own intervention.

There is a specific and underappreciated antidote to decision fatigue that is available between tasks and requires almost no time: brief contact with natural environments. A research team at the University of Melbourne found that a 40-second micro-break involving a glance at a green rooftop garden measurably restored attention and reduced error rates in subsequent tasks compared to equivalent rest breaks spent looking at a concrete surface. The mechanism is the same one described in the Self-Care chapter — involuntary attention, engaged gently by natural environments, restores the depleted directed-attention system without the cognitive overhead of deliberate effort. When you feel your thinking becoming circular, your decisions becoming less discriminating, or your patience with the next email shortening — that is your directed-attention system signaling depletion. Going outside for five minutes is not avoidance. It is the fastest available restoration intervention.[52]

Your physical environment is not a reflection of your mental state. It is a co-creator of it. Shape it accordingly.

How to Build Environmental Design Skills

Environmental design is not a project you finish. It's a practice you maintain — like the garden metaphor from the Self-Care chapter, or the nightly sleep routine from the first. The goal isn't a perfect space. It's a space that is consistently good enough to support rather than undermine everything else.

The Four Drivers work here by reducing the cognitive overhead of environmental maintenance — making the small acts of tending so automatic that they don't require System 2 to remember, decide, or motivate. The environment starts doing the work that willpower was doing badly.

Start Small

The entire apartment doesn't need to be clean. One surface, cleared and maintained, is enough to begin shifting your nervous system's baseline reading of the space. Start there. Stop there. Let it be enough.

- Clear one square foot of your workspace each morning — enough to register a difference, not enough to become a project. The goal is a daily signal, not a deep clean.
- Add one element of calm to your primary space — a plant, a candle, a single meaningful object placed where you'll see it. Not decoration. A deliberate signal to your nervous system that this space is safe and tended.

- Focus on ONE area before moving to the next. Completing one space produces a sense of resolution that scattered improvement across multiple spaces doesn't. Completion is the signal. Get it somewhere before you move on.

Shape Your Environment

The goal is not to create a space you have to maintain through willpower. It's to create a space that maintains itself through design — where putting things away is easier than leaving them out, and where the default behavior is the right behavior.

- Keep your workspace well-lit with natural light where possible. Light is not ambiance — it is a direct input to your circadian system, your alertness, and your mood. Dim environments signal low capacity. Bright environments signal activation. Use that.

- Place a laundry basket exactly where clothes tend to pile up, not where it looks tidiest. You're designing for your actual behavior, not your aspirational behavior. The basket that gets used is the one in the right place.

- Store frequently used items at arm's reach and rarely used items out of sight. Every time you have to search for something, you're paying an attentional tax that compounds across the day. Reduce the search. Reduce the tax.

Link Habits

Environmental maintenance tasks are ideal for habit stacking — they're brief, physically discrete, and produce an immediate visible result. Attach them to existing routines and they cost almost nothing. Left as standalone decisions, they accumulate into the pile that never gets done.

- After your morning coffee — before you open your laptop, before you check your phone — open the blinds. Thirty seconds. The coffee is already automatic. The light catches a ride.

- Pair your circadian light exposure (morning sunlight, open windows) with your first task of the day. You're already doing one; let the other follow automatically.

- Use the 5-4-3-2-1 countdown the moment you notice something out of place. Don't schedule the tidy for later. Later doesn't exist. Count down and move now, while the signal is live.

Celebrate the Wins

Environmental wins disappear into the background the moment they're achieved — a clear desk is just a clear desk. The deliberate pause to notice the difference is how you train your brain to register the improvement as a reward rather than letting it pass unremarked.

- After any act of environmental tending — a cleared surface, an opened blind, a reset desk — pause for five seconds and notice the difference. Not the absence of mess. The presence of calm. Name it. Your nervous system needs to hear that this state is the goal.

- Track one daily environment reset — clearing your desk before bed, setting out your shoes by the door, preparing the coffee station for morning — as a streak. Visible progress on a small, consistent behavior is more motivating than occasional large interventions.

- Treat each tidying session as a practice rep in the skill of environmental stewardship — not housework, but active design of the conditions under which you function best. The frame changes what the behavior means. And what the behavior means is what determines whether you repeat it.

Your Action Steps

1. Start Small

Choose one surface, one space, one object. Not a system. Not an overhaul. One thing:

- "The one space I will focus on first is ____________________ (e.g., my desk, the kitchen counter, the entryway). My minimum daily maintenance of that space is ____________________ (e.g., clear it before bed, tidy it each morning, spend two minutes on it after lunch)."

- "The one element of calm I will add to my primary space is ____________________ (e.g., a plant, natural light, a cleared surface, one object that signals rest or focus). I will place it in ____________________."

- "On days when I have no energy for environmental maintenance, the one thing I will do anyway is ____________________ (e.g., open the blinds, move the laundry off the chair, clear one surface before bed)."

- "I will spend ______________ minutes outside — doorstep, garden, sidewalk — before my first task of the day. Not to exercise. Not to accomplish anything. Just to be briefly in the light, in the air, in something that isn't a screen or a ceiling. This is a nervous system input, not a lifestyle upgrade. Two minutes counts."

2. Shape Your Environment

Design for your actual behavior, not your aspirational behavior:

- "I will place __________________ (laundry basket, shoe rack, charging cable, recycling bin) in __________________ — exactly where the problem currently lives — so the tidy behavior becomes frictionless."

- "I will store __________________ (most-used items) in __________________ (arm's reach location) and move __________________ (rarely used or distracting items) to __________________ (out of sight location)."

- "I will improve the light in __________________ by __________________ (opening blinds, adding a lamp, moving my desk closer to the window) to reduce the low-capacity signal my environment is currently sending."

- "I will place one living plant in __________________ (my workspace, my kitchen, the room I spend the most time in). Not for decoration — as a signal to my nervous system that something alive and growing is sharing the space. If a plant isn't possible, I will find one image of a natural landscape to place where I will see it daily from my desk or chair. The research threshold for this effect is lower than most people assume."

3. Link Habits

Attach environmental maintenance to something that already fires automatically:

- "Immediately after __________________ (morning coffee, brushing teeth, finishing dinner), I will __________________ (open the blinds, clear the counter, reset my desk, put away the one thing that's always out of place)."

- "Every time I ____________________ (leave a room, finish a work block, get up from my desk), I will spend ________ seconds returning ____________________ to its place."

- "When I notice something out of place, I will use ____________________ (5-4-3-2-1, a breath, a single movement) to act on it immediately rather than adding it to a mental list for later."

- "I will pair ____________________ (my first coffee, my lunch break, the end of my workday) with two to five minutes outside, even briefly. I will treat this the way I treat opening the blinds in the Physical Environment chapter — as an environmental input, already decided, that doesn't require a fresh decision each time."

- "I will take a _________ minute walk outside between my two most cognitively demanding administrative blocks. I will do this not as a reward for completing them but as a restoration tool between them. The walk is part of the system, not a break from it. I will treat it the same way I treat the countdown rule — a non-negotiable input to the process rather than an optional addition."

4. Celebrate the Wins

Train your brain to register environmental calm as a reward, not just the absence of chaos:

- "After I tidy or reset my space, I will pause for five seconds and notice ____________________ (the cleared surface, the open light, the reduced background noise) and say to myself: ____________________ (e.g., 'This is what support feels like,' 'I built this')."

- "I will track my daily environment reset — ____________________ (clearing my desk, setting out tomorrow's items, a five-minute tidy) — by marking ____________________ every day I complete it."

- "If I maintain my environmental reset habit for ________ days in a row, I will reward myself with ____________________."

My Environment Commitment

Write it down. Name the space. Name the action. Keep it small enough that you'll actually do it every day.

New Behavior:
What, specifically, will you do? In which space?

The Setup:
How will you physically arrange your space to make this easier than not doing it?

The Trigger:
I will do this immediately before/after I:

The Celebration:
I will acknowledge my success by:

Becoming You

At first, environment feels like a background issue:

I should clean up more. I should organize my desk. I should make my space feel calmer.

'Should' doesn't survive fatigue, distraction, or the endless internal negotiation about whether now is really the right time. A supportive environment doesn't arrive through occasional deep cleans or weekend overhauls. It grows through repeated, unremarkable acts. Clearing one counter before bed. Opening the blinds when you wake up. Putting the shoes back where they belong. Moving the one thing that's always in the wrong place.

Each act is small enough to be invisible and significant enough to shift your nervous system's baseline reading of the space. Not dramatically. A fraction. But fractions compound. And a nervous system that has spent a day in a calm, ordered environment arrives at the evening different than one that has spent the same day in chaos and friction.

At first System 2 does all the work — the reminders, the decisions, the deliberate choices to tidy when every impulse says do it later. Over time, the repetitions accumulate. Each small act lowers the threshold for the next one. Until clearing the counter before bed is simply what happens at the end of the day, the way brushing your teeth is simply what happens.

System 2 passes the baton to System 1. And what once felt like maintenance becomes just... how you live.

You are no longer at the mercy of your surroundings, reacting to chaos you never chose. You are someone who shapes your spaces to match your values — who creates environments that restore rather than deplete, that support rather than sabotage. The physical world around you becomes a quiet source of strength rather than a constant drain.

Daniel got there. Not through a weekend overhaul or a perfectly organized apartment. Through moving a pair of shoes and opening the blinds, repeated until it removed a thousand tiny pebbles from his shoes and he could finally walk forward unburdened.

So can you.

Life Administration

Skill #6: The Systems That Keep Your Life Moving

"You do not rise to the level of your goals. You fall to the level of your systems."
— James Clear

Jennifer

Jennifer's desk was a graveyard of unopened envelopes. Utility bills. Insurance notices. Something from the bank she hadn't dared open, its window envelope face-down as if that made it less real. Her email inbox showed over 3,000 unread messages — most of them junk, but some carrying the quiet, specific weight of things she already knew she'd failed to do. Appointments she'd missed. Forms she'd promised to return. People she owed responses to.

She told herself she'd catch up this weekend. This weekend became next weekend. Weekends came and went, swallowed whole by the fog of her depression, which had a particular talent for making the manageable feel insurmountable and the urgent feel abstract.

Each ignored task carried a small cost. A late fee that arrived without warning. A forgotten appointment that had to be rescheduled with an apology. A reminder silenced and never revisited, sliding silently off the edge of her awareness. Nothing catastrophic on its own — but together they built a steady, low-frequency hum of dread that sat just beneath the surface of every day, never fully quiet. When her phone buzzed with another alert she couldn't face, she'd silence it and then sit staring at the middle distance, gripped by the particular shame of someone convinced they were failing at the basic maintenance of being an adult. Not the extraordinary parts. The ordinary ones. The parts everyone else seemed to manage without thinking.

One afternoon, a friend came over and sat with her at the desk. Not to fix anything. Just to be there while Jennifer opened one envelope. A utility bill. Overdue, but not catastrophically so. Payable, with a phone call.

The world didn't end. More than that — something released. A pressure she'd been carrying for so long she'd stopped registering it as a weight, the way you stop hearing the hum of a refrigerator until it finally switches off.

The next day, she answered one email. Not three thousand. One. A week later, she set a single calendar reminder for an appointment she'd been avoiding. Tiny actions, each of them objectively unimpressive. But each one chipped away at something larger than the pile on her desk — the story she'd been telling herself about who she was. Someone who couldn't cope. Someone who'd lost the thread entirely.

Slowly, the pile shrank. The inbox became less menacing. She began, cautiously and without much fanfare, to trust herself again.

Life administration was never going to be joyful — that was never the point. But it became manageable.

And manageable, she discovered, was everything.

Life Administration Quiz

Before we get into specifics, take two minutes to answer these questions. Answer honestly so you get a sense of how this past week has actually been for you.

This past week, how satisfied were you with your ability to manage day-to-day responsibilities?

⓪ Very dissatisfied ① Dissatisfied ② Fairly satisfied ③ Very satisfied

When did you last wash laundry, bed sheets, pillowcases, or towels?

⓪ Over 2 weeks ago ① Over 1 week ago ② A few days ago ③ This week

This past week, how stressed were you about paying bills or staying on top of finances?

⓪ Very stressed ① Somewhat stressed ② A little stressed ③ Not at all stressed

How competent did you feel in managing your life administration this past week?

⓪ Very incompetent ① Somewhat incompetent ② Fairly competent ③ Very competent

How consistently did you manage your medications or supplements this past week?

⓪ Not at all ① Somewhat ② Fairly well ③ Consistently

Your Score: __________ (Total: 0–15)

- If 0–5: Start by centralizing your to-dos and key dates in one place. One list. One calendar. The goal is visibility, not perfection.
- If 6–10: Strengthen your systems for tracking and follow-through. Identify the two or three tasks that cause the most stress and build a specific system for each.
- If 11–15: Maintain efficiency and refine for simplicity. Good systems should require less effort over time, not more. If yours are getting heavier, simplify.

What Life Administration Actually Is

Life administration is the unglamorous plumbing of a functioning existence. It is the quiet, uncelebrated work that keeps everything else from collapsing in on itself: paying bills, managing calendars, renewing documents, handling the inbox, tracking the prescriptions, maintaining the household. None of it is thrilling. All of it is load-bearing.

Think of it as the scaffolding beneath everything else you're trying to build. When it's solid, you don't notice it. You're too busy doing the actual work. When it's rotting, you notice nothing else — because the creaking and swaying consume all available attention. A missed payment, a forgotten appointment, a tax deadline that arrives like a surprise, a prescription that ran out three days ago — these aren't just inconveniences. They are avoidable stress events that activate System 1, flood it with urgency, and crowd out the System 2 capacity that the rest of your life depends on.

Done well, life admin produces the opposite effect: a stable backdrop of 'things are handled.' This is not a small thing. It frees System 2 from the constant cognitive overhead of tracking what's slipping, what's overdue, what might be about to become a crisis — and redirects that capacity toward the thinking, planning, and creating that actually moves your life forward.

Life admin spans four domains, each carrying its own cognitive and emotional load:

- Financial upkeep — bills, budgeting, tracking expenses, avoiding the cascade that starts with one missed payment.
- Time management — calendars, reminders, scheduling, the invisible architecture that determines whether you show up or disappear.

- Household management — maintenance, repairs, keeping essentials stocked, the physical infrastructure of daily life.
- Digital organization — the inbox, the files, the passwords, the cloud storage that becomes a digital archaeological dig if left unattended.

None of these domains are glamorous. All of them, kept in reasonable order, are invisible. And that invisibility is the goal: a life admin system that works is one you don't have to think about. A life admin system that doesn't work is one you can't stop thinking about.

Why Life Admin Is Infrastructure, Not Busywork

Life administration is not the alternative to doing important things. It is the foundation on which important things become possible. Every loose end, overdue obligation, and unresolved administrative task sends a continuous signal to your nervous system: something is slipping. System 1 reads disorganization as threat. System 2, operating on the degraded cognitive resources that System 1's background vigilance leaves behind, has less capacity for the thinking that actually matters. Both systems sputter when the scaffolding is rotting.

The Cost of Neglect

- Cognitive clutter: Your brain is simultaneously tracking what's overdue, what's coming, and what might be about to become a crisis — bandwidth that could be used for anything else.
- Chronic micro-stress: Every unchecked task is a low-level cortisol stimulus. Multiply by twenty tasks and the load becomes significant. Multiply by twenty tasks over twenty days and you have chronic low-level panic.

- Decision fatigue: Without systems, every administrative task requires fresh effort. The fifteenth decision of the day costs more than the first, regardless of its actual complexity.[31]

- Avoidance loops: Disorganization produces overwhelm. Overwhelm produces procrastination. Procrastination increases disorganization. The loop tightens until a friend sits with you and helps you open one envelope.

- Destabilized habits: When the administrative scaffolding is shaky, even well-established habits in other domains become harder to maintain. The structure that holds the whole system up is cracked.

The Payoff of Well-Maintained Systems

- Cognitive clarity: When things are handled, your brain stops tracking them. The freed bandwidth is immediately available for whatever actually requires your attention.

- Reduced baseline stress: A life admin system that works lowers the chronic low-frequency hum of 'what am I forgetting' that Jennifer's story describes. This is not a minor improvement. It is a measurable reduction in allostatic load.

- Frictionless habits: Good systems automate the behaviors that matter — the bill paid automatically, the appointment already in the calendar, the prescription refilled before it runs out. Automation is the highest form of habit design.

- More energy for what matters: Fewer fires to fight means more bandwidth for the people, projects, and pursuits that make the administrative maintenance worth doing in the first place.

- Long-term resilience: Stable systems make life predictable in the best sense — anchored, manageable, and supportive of everything built on top of them.

Life Administration and Long-Term Mental Health

The relationship between life administration and mental health runs in both directions — and it operates through mechanisms that are more specific and more powerful than most people recognize.

Administrative neglect is a reliable cortisol generator. Each unresolved task, unread bill, and unchecked obligation sends a low-level threat signal to the nervous system. Individually, each signal is minor. Cumulatively, across a day, a week, a month of accumulating administrative backlog, they produce allostatic load — the biological wear of chronic stress exposure — that predisposes the nervous system to anxiety, depression, and reduced resilience under subsequent stressors. You are not anxious *because* you have a personality prone to anxiety. You are anxious because your brain is tracking forty-seven unresolved obligations and treating each one as a potential threat.

Depression makes administrative collapse particularly vicious because it attacks the exact capacities needed to address it. Motivation, executive function, the ability to initiate action on tasks that feel pointless or overwhelming — these are precisely what depression degrades. The unopened envelope pile grows not because you are lazy or irresponsible, but because the neurobiological state of depression has reduced the cognitive and motivational resources available to address it. The pile then becomes evidence of failure, which worsens shame, which worsens depression, which further reduces the capacity to address the pile. The loop tightens.

This is why the friend sitting with Jennifer while she opens one envelope is not a trivial detail. It is the mechanism of the intervention. Administrative tasks that feel impossible alone become possible with witnessed, non-judgmental presence — because the shame that makes them impossible is a social emotion that responds to social correction. You cannot shame yourself into addressing your shame. You can, with help, take one action that demonstrates the loop can be broken.

Good life administration is, in this sense, a form of preventive mental health care. Systems that handle the administrative load automatically — the autopay, the calendar reminder, the prescription refill scheduled in advance — remove the chronic cortisol stimulus before it accumulates into something harder to address. The goal is not an organized life for its own sake. The goal is a nervous system that isn't spending its limited resources tracking things that could be handled by a system.

How to Build Life Administration Skills

Life administration is the non-negotiable most directly undermined by depression. The tasks feel pointless. The pile feels insurmountable. The shame of how far behind you've fallen makes starting feel worse than not starting. The Four Drivers don't fix that feeling. They lower the initiation cost until the action happens despite the feeling. That's the whole game.

The goal isn't an organized life. It's a first action small enough that the resistance can't match it. One email. One envelope. One calendar entry. The resistance is strong. Make the action smaller.

Start Small

The task isn't to clear the inbox. The task is to open one email. The task isn't to organize the finances. The task is to pay one bill. Make the unit as small as possible and hold the boundary there. The resistance is calibrated to the whole pile. The action only has to be one item.

- Spend two minutes each morning on one email folder — not the whole inbox, one folder. Small enough that the dread doesn't have time to build before you've already started.

- Complete one administrative task per day — one bill paid, one form filed, one appointment scheduled. One. The momentum from consistent small completions builds more reliably than occasional heroic clearing sessions.
- Master one organizational tool before adding another. One calendar. One task list. One system that you actually use, imperfectly, beats five systems you maintain for a week and abandon.
- Block time in your schedule for intentional life administration.

Shape Your Environment

Administrative tasks die in the gap between thinking of them and having the tools to do them. Close that gap. Everything you need to handle an administrative task should be immediately accessible the moment the task occurs to you. Friction is the enemy. Eliminate it by design.

- Keep a visible task list in your primary workspace — not in an app you have to open, somewhere you can't not see it. What stays visible stays manageable. What disappears into apps and notes gets forgotten and accumulates.
- Store bill-paying supplies together in one place — checkbook, stamps, envelopes, pen. One location. If paying a bill requires assembling four objects from four places, you won't pay the bill. If it requires reaching into one drawer, you will.
- Block a fixed weekly time for administrative work in your calendar — the same day, the same time, every week. The decision to do admin work should never need to be made again. It's already made. The same day every week/month.

Link Habits

Administrative tasks are brief enough to catch a ride on almost any existing habit. Making coffee literally takes three minutes. Unloading the dishwasher takes no more than 5 minutes. Let them happen together until they become the same habit.

- After making your morning coffee — before opening anything else — open your task list and identify the one administrative task you will complete today. Not all of them. One. The coffee is already automatic. The task identification catches a ride.

- Pair tedious administrative tasks with something genuinely enjoyable — a specific playlist, a good coffee, a walk immediately after. You're not bribing yourself. You're training your brain to associate the hard thing with a reliable reward that follows it.

- Use the 5-4-3-2-1 countdown the moment an administrative task occurs to you. Don't add it to a list for later. Count down and start the task before the avoidance loop can complete. The longer the gap between thinking of the task and starting it, the less likely it is to happen.

Celebrate the Wins

Administrative tasks produce no creative value and receive little external recognition (if any). The envelope paid disappears into the system. The email answered generates another email. The calendar updated looks the same as it did before. The internal acknowledgment is therefore your only reinforcement signal — and it needs to be deliberate, because nothing else will provide it.

- After completing any administrative task — however small — say 'done' out loud or mark it off visibly. This is not a performance. It is a dopaminergic signal. Your brain needs to hear that the task is complete and that completion is a good outcome. Tell it.

- Track daily completions rather than the overall backlog. The backlog is a measure of the past. Completions are a measure of the present. Track what you're doing, not what you haven't done.

- Treat each administrative completion as a practice rep for the skill of follow-through — not a chore survived, but evidence that you can initiate, execute, and complete. That evidence accumulates into the self-trust that Jennifer rebuilt, one opened envelope at a time.

Your Action Steps

1. Start Small

Name the single smallest administrative action you are willing to take today:

- "The one administrative task I will complete today, no matter what, is ____________________ (e.g., pay one bill, answer one email, file one document, schedule one appointment)."

- "The administrative area causing me the most background stress is ____________________. The smallest possible first action I could take on it is ____________________."

- "On days when I have no capacity for administrative work, the one thing I will do anyway is ____________________ (e.g., open my task list and look at it, delete five emails, check one item off the list)."

2. Shape Your Environment

Design for accessibility: the task that requires the least effort to start is the task that gets done:

- "I will create a visible task list in ________________ (my planner, a whiteboard, a sticky note on my desk, a dedicated app I actually check) and review it every ________________."
- "I will store my bill-paying supplies — ________________ — together in ________________ so paying a bill never requires assembling anything."
- "I will block ________________ (day and time) in my calendar as my weekly administrative time. This decision is made. It doesn't need to be made again."

3. Link Habits

Attach administrative tasks to something that already happens automatically:

- "Immediately after ________________ (morning coffee, sitting down at my desk, finishing lunch), I will ________________ (open my task list, answer one email, complete one administrative task I've been avoiding)."
- "I will pair ________________ (my most avoided administrative task) with ________________ (a specific enjoyable activity that follows it) so my brain learns to associate it with a reliable reward."
- "When an administrative task occurs to me, I will count ________________ out loud and start it before I finish counting, rather than adding it to a list for later."

4. Celebrate the Wins

Give your brain the signal that administrative completion is a reward, not just a relief:

- "After completing any administrative task, I will __________________ (say 'done' out loud, check it off visibly, take five seconds to acknowledge it) to register the completion as a positive outcome."
- "I will track my daily administrative completions in __________________ (a notebook, a habit tracker, a tally on my task list) — counting what I'm doing, not what remains."
- "If I complete one administrative task every day for _______ days, I will reward myself with __________________."

My Life Administration Commitment

Write it down. Name the specific task. Keep the scope small enough that not doing it would require more effort than doing it.

New Behavior:
What, specifically, will you do? (One task. Name it.)

The Setup:
How will you make this task immediately accessible when the trigger fires?

The Trigger:
I will do this immediately before/after I:

The Celebration:
I will acknowledge my completion by:

Becoming You

At first, life administration feels like a nagging accusation:

I should pay those bills. I should answer those emails. I should finally organize my calendar.

'Should' rarely survives exhaustion, depression, or the comforting illusion that tomorrow will be different. Real administrative competence doesn't arrive through heroic weekend clearing sessions or a perfect new system. It grows through repeated, ordinary, often boring acts. One bill paid on time. One email answered before the pile grows by ten more. One calendar entry that means you show up rather than forget. Each small completion is a message to your nervous system: this is manageable. I can do this. Something is handled.

At first System 2 does all the work — the reminders, the lists, the effortful initiation of tasks that feel pointless or shameful or overwhelming. It is effortful. For people managing depression, it can feel nearly impossible. But each completion — however small — lays down a thin layer of evidence that the loop can be interrupted. And evidence accumulates.

Over time, System 2 passes the baton to System 1. Checking the task list becomes what you do after coffee. Paying the bill becomes what you do on Tuesday. The administrative rhythm becomes part of the structure of your week rather than a separate decision that requires fresh motivation every time.

You are no longer someone playing perpetual catch-up, living with the low-frequency hum of things slipping. You are someone whose systems work — quietly, imperfectly, invisibly — in the background of a life that has enough structure to hold. The scaffolding is solid. You can build on it.

Jennifer got there. Not through a complete system overhaul or a perfect inbox. Through opening one envelope with a friend beside her, then another, until she trusted herself.

Slowly but steadily she found freedom through structure.

So can you.

Community & Belonging

Skill #7: The Human Lifeline

"Connection is why we're here. It's what gives purpose and meaning to our lives."
— Brené Brown

Lusia

Lusia kept a sticky note on her fridge that read, *Reach out.*

It had been there for months, curling at the corners from the steam of a hundred reheated meals, yellowing slightly at the edges. More accusation than inspiration. She'd stopped really seeing it, the way you stop seeing anything that's been in the same place long enough.

She told herself she should connect more. Call a friend. Make the effort. But *should* is no match for inertia, especially when inertia has a comfortable couch and three unwatched seasons of something on Netflix. Most evenings ended exactly that way — the glow of a screen, a glass of something, and the quiet hum of something she didn't quite have a word for yet.

The isolation had crept in gradually, the way most things do. A job change that dissolved a social ecosystem overnight. A breakup that redistributed their mutual friends in ways nobody formally announced. A pandemic that rebranded staying home as responsible citizenship. By the time she looked up and noticed, loneliness had become her default state — not the dramatic, cinematic kind that announces itself in tears, but the low-grade ache of realizing, at 7pm on a Wednesday, that she hadn't had a real conversation in over a week.

She knew, in the abstract, that isolation was bad for her. She'd read the articles. She knew what the research said about loneliness and cortisol and cardiovascular health. Knowing didn't fix it. It never does.

The first step was almost embarrassingly small: she texted an old coworker. Just Hey, thinking of you. Seven words, no punctuation, sent before she could talk herself out of it. The reply came back warm and immediate, and something in her chest loosened — a tension so familiar she'd stopped registering it as tension. She tried again the following week: she said yes to a neighborhood dinner she would normally have declined with a plausible excuse. She arrived awkward, left early, and still — something had shifted. A laugh shared over bad wine. A story that reminded her she had stories worth telling.

She built scaffolding around the fragile new habit. After Sunday morning coffee — already a non-negotiable ritual — she would text one person. Just one. The coffee made it feel smaller. The routine made it automatic.

Weeks became months. A standing Tuesday call with her sister. Monthly brunch with two neighbors. The occasional walk with a coworker who turned out to be funnier than she'd expected. Each small act of connection made the next one fractionally easier, the way a path through tall grass gets clearer each time someone walks it.

One day she noticed the sticky note was gone — she'd taken it down without ceremony, without even registering it as a milestone. She no longer needed the reminder.

She simply had people now. And that changed everything.

Community & Belonging Quiz

Before we get into specifics, take two minutes to answer these questions. Answer honestly so you get a sense of how this past week has actually been for you.

This past week, how satisfied were you with your sense of community and belonging?

⓪ Very dissatisfied ① Dissatisfied ② Fairly satisfied ③ Very satisfied

How often did you spend time in person with people in your community?

⓪ Never ① 1–2 times ② 3–4 times ③ Every day

How did your interactions this week break down: online vs. in person?

⓪ All online ① Mostly online ② Mostly in person ③ All in person

How comfortable did you feel bringing your full, authentic self to your interactions?

⓪ Not comfortable ① Somewhat comfortable ② Fairly comfortable ③ Very comfortable

How often did you feel that people genuinely had your back?

⓪ Never ① Occasionally ② Often ③ Always

Your Score: __________ (Total: 0–15)

- If 0–5: Start with one safe, honest connection. Quality before quantity. Depth before breadth.
- If 6–10: Increase consistency and begin deepening existing relationships rather than expanding the network.
- If 11–15: Maintain what you have and actively nurture it. Connection erodes without attention.

What Community & Belonging Actually Are

Community and belonging are not measured by your contact list or your follower count. They are about something older, deeper, and more visceral: the felt sense of safety, acceptance, and mutual care that comes from being truly known by another person.

From an evolutionary standpoint, belonging was not a preference. It was a survival mechanism. For most of human history, we lived and died with our tribe. They fed us, defended us, and kept us warm when the nights turned dangerous. To be cast out was not a social inconvenience — it was a death sentence, as certain as a predator's teeth. Our nervous system has not forgotten this. The same circuitry that once scanned the savanna for rustling grass now scans our inbox for who hasn't replied — triggering the same hormonal cascade that once followed the sound of approaching danger. The threat has changed. Biology hasn't.

Belonging is an emotional home — a place where we are not merely seen but recognized, wanted, and missed. The kind of place where we know: *they would notice if I didn't come back*. Without it, we don't just feel lonely. We feel morally unhinged — like actors without a stage, performing for no one. And the body registers this as a threat. Chronic loneliness is associated with elevated cortisol, persistent inflammation, and a nervous system rewired for hypervigilance rather than trust.

Social connection exists in layers, each serving a different biological need:

- Inner circle — family, close friends, partners — who hold our history and our vulnerabilities and still move closer rather than away.
- Affinity groups — communities built around shared values, interests, or goals: the climbing partners, the choir, the fellow parents on the sidelines.

- Wider networks — looser ties that still anchor us in a larger web of meaning and mutual recognition such as UPS drivers, grocery store clerks, dog-walking neighbors, etc.

A healthy social life draws from all three. Inner circles provide emotional shelter. Affinity groups supply identity and shared mission. Wider networks connect us to the unpredictable richness of the world beyond our immediate experience.

System 1 treats belonging as safety — because for most of human evolutionary history, it was. System 2 is the part of us that can recognize this drive, work with it deliberately, and take steps to build connection even when anxiety or exhaustion or old rejection wounds make the instinct to withdraw feel compelling. Belonging is not a fixed state we either have or don't. It's a skill. And like every skill in this book, it gets better with practice.

Why Belonging Is a Biological Need

Loneliness is not a mood. It's a physiological state with measurable consequences. Research on social isolation — most notably a 2010 meta-analysis by Julianne Holt-Lunstad covering 300,000 participants — established that chronic loneliness is as damaging to long-term health as smoking fifteen cigarettes a day[32] — not as metaphor, but as a quantifiable increase in mortality risk. Our nervous system treats social exclusion as a threat to survival, because for most of human evolutionary history, it was.

The Cost of Neglect

- Disconnection in company: Feeling invisible or peripheral even when surrounded by people — the loneliness of being unseen rather than alone.

- Surface-level interactions: Conversations that stay in the shallows, leaving a vague dissatisfaction that's hard to name.

- Reluctance to ask for help: Silent suffering driven by the fear of being burdensome — which compounds isolation by making it invisible.
- Social fatigue: Interactions that drain rather than replenish, because they require performance rather than authentic presence.
- Persistent outsider feeling: The low-grade sense of being adjacent to a community rather than inside it.

The Payoff of Genuine Connection

- Emotional resilience: Strong social bonds are the most robust buffer against stress in the psychological literature. Connection doesn't eliminate difficulty — it makes it survivable.
- Physical health: Supportive relationships reduce inflammatory markers, regulate cortisol, and measurably improve immune function and cardiovascular outcomes.
- Cognitive vitality: Engaged social life stimulates memory, empathy, and perspective-taking in ways that solitary activity cannot replicate.
- Meaning and purpose: A sense of place in something larger than yourself is one of the most consistent predictors of psychological well-being across cultures and across the lifespan.
- Daily joy: Laughter, shared ritual, and the ordinary pleasure of being known — these are not luxuries. They are what makes a life feel like a life.

Community, Belonging, and Long-Term Mental Health

The relationship between social connection and mental health is bidirectional — and the mechanisms are more specific than most people realize.

Genuine connection triggers the release of oxytocin, which reduces amygdala reactivity and lowers the physiological stress response.[33] It stimulates dopamine pathways associated with reward and motivation. Even casual positive social contact — a brief conversation, a moment of shared laughter, a text that lands warmly — produces measurable neurochemical shifts that reduce baseline anxiety and support mood regulation. These are not trivial effects. They are the nervous system doing exactly what it was designed to do in the presence of safe others.

Here is the vicious loop that chronic isolation creates: loneliness activates the threat response. The threat response elevates cortisol and inflammatory cytokines. Chronic inflammation and cortisol dysregulation are directly associated with depression, anxiety, and PTSD symptom severity. Depression and anxiety reduce motivation to seek social contact. Reduced social contact feeds loneliness. The loop tightens.

Cacioppo's research adds a further layer: chronically lonely people don't just feel more threatened — they become more hypervigilant, more likely to interpret ambiguous social signals as hostile,[34] and more likely to withdraw preemptively to avoid anticipated rejection. The nervous system, trying to protect you from further pain, ends up building the prison it was trying to avoid.

From a systems perspective: isolation leaves System 1 running paranoid and defensive, scanning for social threat in every ambiguous interaction. System 2 — the part that could recognize the loop, challenge the interpretations, and take deliberate steps toward connection — is running on a depleted tank. The very cognitive resources needed to build community are eroded by the absence of it.

Community is not an accessory to mental health treatment. For many people, it is the treatment.

How to Build Community & Belonging Skills

Most people who struggle with community know exactly what they should do. Text a friend. Join a group. Show up. The obstacle isn't information — it's the weight of anxiety, past rejection, and a nervous system that has learned to treat vulnerability as dangerous.

The Four Drivers work here not by overcoming that fear with willpower — that approach has a poor track record — but by lowering the stakes of each individual act until System 1 stops treating connection as threat and starts treating it as habit. Small. Repeated. Safe enough to try again.

There is one context for social connection that the research consistently highlights and that everyday life consistently underutilizes: the outdoors. Side-by-side activity in natural settings — walking together, working in a garden, hiking, playing in a park — produces a quality of social bonding that face-to-face, indoors interaction tends not to replicate. Part of the mechanism is attentional: when you're walking beside someone, the shared forward orientation and the continuous mild stimulation of the environment reduce the self-consciousness and performance pressure that indoor conversations can carry. Part of it is physiological: both people are getting the cortisol-reducing, autonomically-regulating effects of the natural environment simultaneously, which lowers defensive arousal and creates the conditions in which authentic disclosure feels safer. Research on the "soft fascination" of natural environments suggests that they occupy enough attention to quiet the vigilance loop without demanding enough attention to crowd out conversation. The result is that people talk more openly, listen more generously, and feel more connected after an hour walking outside together than after an equivalent hour seated across from each other indoors.[56]

This doesn't require elaborate planning. Suggest a walk instead of a coffee. Take a phone call while moving through a park. Join or start an outdoor group activity — a hiking group, a community garden, a regular outdoor game. The connection happens in the doing, not in creating the perfect conditions for it.

Start Small

The goal isn't an impressive social life. The goal is a first rep that doesn't trigger the retreat response. Small enough that it's hard to talk yourself out of it before you've done it.

- Greet one colleague or neighbor each day by name. Recognition is the entry point to belonging — and it asks almost nothing of either person.
- Send one short message of appreciation or check-in to one person this week. Not a scheduled call. Not a vulnerable conversation. One text. Low stakes, high signal: you're still there.
- Deepen one existing relationship rather than trying to build new ones from scratch. You already have the raw material. Use it.

Shape Your Environment

Anxiety lives in the gap between intention and action. Environment design closes that gap by making the decision before the anxiety has a chance to make it for you.

- Keep a visible list of three to five people you want to stay in touch with — on your wall, your fridge, or your phone's home screen. What you can see, you act on. What you have to remember, you forget.

- Place thank-you cards and stamps somewhere visible. Spontaneous connection is more likely when the friction to act on it is near zero.

- Join one group that meets at a fixed time and place on a regular basis. Let the calendar make the choice so your anxiety doesn't have to. Consistency of the environment is the fastest route to consistency of behavior.

Link Habits

The social behaviors most likely to survive anxiety and low motivation are the ones that don't require a decision in the moment. Attach them to something that already runs on autopilot and let System 1 carry the load.

- After your morning coffee — or whatever ritual already anchors your morning — send one text to check in on someone. One. The ritual lowers the activation energy. The habit does the rest.

- Pair a walk or workout with a phone call to a friend or family member. You're spending the time anyway. Let the connection ride along.

- Use the 5-4-3-2-1 countdown to initiate a conversation with someone new before System 1 generates an exit strategy. The countdown interrupts the avoidance loop before it completes.

Celebrate the Wins

For someone whose nervous system has learned to associate social contact with risk, the celebration step is especially important — and especially easy to skip. Don't skip it. The brief moment of acknowledgment after a positive interaction fires a dopaminergic signal that tells your threat-detection system: that was safe. That is worth doing again. Over time, those signals accumulate into a new default.

- After any act of connection — a text sent, a call made, a yes given to an invitation — pause and acknowledge it. 'I did that.' That's enough. You're not performing gratitude. You're updating the nervous system's threat assessment.

- Track your weekly social touchpoints. Not to optimize them — just to make them visible. What gets measured gets noticed. What gets noticed gets repeated.

- Treat each interaction as a practice rep for the skills of empathy, presence, and genuine communication — not a test of whether you're likable. You're practicing, not auditioning.

Your Action Steps

1. Start Small

Make the first step small enough that anxiety can't reasonably object:

- "The one social act I will do this week no matter what is ____________________ (e.g., text one person, say hi to a neighbor, reply to a message I've been avoiding)."

- "The person I most want to reconnect with is ____________________. My first step toward that reconnection is ____________________ (e.g., a text, a voice memo, a short email)."

- "Instead of trying to build a whole social life at once, I will focus only on deepening my relationship with ____________________ this month."

2. Shape Your Environment

Design your environment to close the gap between intention and action:

- "I will keep a list of ____________________ people I want to stay in touch with in ____________________ (on my fridge, in my phone notes, on a sticky note by my desk) so I see them regularly."
- "I will join ____________________ (a class, a group, a club, a recurring event) that meets at ____________________ on ____________________ so the schedule makes the decision for me."
- "I will place ____________________ (thank-you cards, my phone, a journal) in ____________________ so that reaching out requires less effort than not reaching out."

3. Link Habits

Attach connection to something that already runs automatically:

- "Immediately after ____________________ (my morning coffee, my workout, my lunch break), I will ____________________ (text one person, make a short call, send a voice message)."
- "I will pair my ____________________ (walk, commute, workout) with calling ____________________ so that movement and connection happen at the same time."
- "When I feel the urge to cancel or withdraw, I will use ____________________ (5-4-3-2-1, a breath, a single text) to interrupt the avoidance loop before it completes."
- "I will move one existing social connection — a regular call, a weekly check-in, a standing catch-up — outside. I will

propose a walk to ________________ instead of a sit-down. If they can't, I'll still take the call while walking. The outdoor context is the intervention; the conversation is already happening."

4. Celebrate the Wins

Give your nervous system the signal that connection was safe and worth repeating:

- "After any act of reaching out — however small — I will take five seconds to say to myself: ________________ (e.g., 'I showed up,' 'That counts,' 'I'm building this')."
- "I will track my social touchpoints by ________________ (marking a calendar, keeping a note in my phone, a habit tracking app) to make my progress visible."
- "If I maintain my connection habit for ______ days in a row, I will reward myself with ________________."

My Community & Belonging Commitment

Write it down. Specific. Simple. Small enough that anxiety can't talk you out of it before you've done it.

New Behavior:
What, specifically, will you do? (Keep it small enough to feel safe.)

The Setup:
How will you prepare your environment so connection is easier than avoidance?

The Trigger:
I will do this immediately before/after I:

The Celebration:
I will acknowledge my success by:

Becoming You

At first, belonging feels like a wish:

I should connect more. I should reach out. I should make more of an effort.

But 'should' is no match for inertia, anxiety, or the memory of a time when reaching out didn't go well. Real belonging doesn't arrive through a single brave conversation or a perfectly curated social life. It grows through repeated, ordinary, almost invisible acts. A text sent on a Sunday morning. A yes given to an invitation you would usually decline. A walk taken with someone instead of alone. Each act sends a signal to the nervous system: this was safe. This is what people do. This is who I am.

At first System 2 does all the work — the reminders, the awkward first steps, the deliberate choices to show up when every impulse says stay home. It feels effortful. Sometimes it is effortful. But the repetitions accumulate. Each connection lays down a thin layer of neural infrastructure — a slightly lower threat response, a slightly higher baseline of trust — until reaching out becomes less of a decision and more of a reflex.

System 2 passes the baton to System 1. And what once required courage becomes just... *Tuesday.*

You stop seeing yourself as someone trying to be less lonely. You start seeing yourself as someone who is woven into a web of care — not because you performed it into existence, but because you showed up enough times that it became real. The identity isn't claimed. It's built, one unremarkable interaction at a time.

Lusia got there. Not through a single act of courage. Through a text sent on a Sunday morning after coffee, repeated until it became the kind of person she was. So can you.

Meaning & Purpose

Skill #8: The Compass for Your Life

"The meaning of life is to find your gift. The purpose of life is to give it away."
— Pablo Picasso

Paul

Paul had done everything right — or at least everything he'd been told was right. Top of his class. Law review. A respectable firm job secured before the ink on his diploma was dry. His parents beamed when they introduced him at family gatherings: our son, the lawyer. His LinkedIn profile glowed like a storefront window, curated and impressive and entirely accurate.

And yet.

On Monday mornings, Paul sat at his desk staring at contracts that felt like an endless loop of déjà vu — redlines, revisions, billable hours logged with the quiet efficiency of someone performing a task in a dream. His chest tightened when he looked at the clock. Not from the workload. From the creeping, persistent suspicion that he was spending his one life on something that wasn't quite his own — wearing a suit that fit perfectly and belonged to someone else entirely.

The thought surfaced during late nights at the office, long after the partners had gone home and the floor had gone quiet. Is this it? He told himself he should be grateful. Plenty of people would take this stability without a second thought. And still the unease grew — not into hatred, never that, but into something more corrosive: the feeling that he was using his tools to build someone else's house, year after year, billing in six-minute increments.

One evening, walking home after a twelve-hour day, he passed a legal aid clinic two blocks from his apartment — a place he'd walked past dozens of times without really seeing it. Through the glass he watched young attorneys helping families navigate paperwork they could never have managed alone. It looked messy. Loud. Nothing like the clean, climate-controlled precision of his firm. But it looked alive and meaningful in a way his work hadn't felt in years.

He stood on the pavement longer than he meant to. Then he walked inside and asked if they needed volunteers.

The first session was humbling. He was slower than the staff attorneys, uncertain about procedures he'd never encountered at the firm, quietly startled by how much he didn't know. But when a family walked out with what they'd come in for — relief moving visibly across their faces like weather clearing — Paul felt something he hadn't felt in years. Not the satisfaction of billing a strong hour. Something older and simpler than that. Something that felt, distantly, like usefulness.

He went back the following week. And the week after that.

He didn't quit his job, not yet. But the center of gravity in his life had shifted — subtly, irreversibly. Purpose, he was learning, wasn't a destination you arrived at. It was a direction you practiced your way into, one Tuesday evening at a time.

Meaning & Purpose Quiz

Before we get into specifics, take two minutes to answer these questions. Answer honestly so you get a sense of how this past week has actually been for you.

This past week, how satisfied were you with your sense of purpose?

⓪ Very dissatisfied ① Dissatisfied ② Fairly satisfied
③ Very satisfied

How competent did you feel in living in alignment with your core values?

⓪ Very incompetent ① Somewhat incompetent ② Fairly competent
③ Very competent

How many days did you feel your life is heading in a positive direction?

⓪ Never ① 1–2 days ② 3–4 days ③ Every day

How often did you feel you made a meaningful contribution to others?

⓪ Never ① Occasionally ② Often ③ Every day

How often did you feel valued or recognized by the people around you?

⓪ Never ① Occasionally ② Often ③ Every day

Your Score: __________ (Total: 0–15)

- If 0–5: Begin with self-reflection to clarify what actually matters to you — not what should matter, what does. Start there.
- If 6–10: Align daily actions with your emerging sense of purpose. One values-aligned choice per day is enough to begin shifting the direction of travel.
- If 11–15: Deepen and expand. Purpose that stays contained within one domain eventually stagnates. Look for where it wants to grow.

What Meaning & Purpose Actually Are

Meaning and purpose are related but not identical, and the distinction matters.

Meaning is retrospective: it's the sense, looking back, that what you've done has counted for something — that your struggles had a point, your relationships left a mark, your efforts were not wasted. Purpose, on the other hand, is prospective: it's the orientation that guides what you do next. You can have meaning without clear purpose (a life well-lived that wasn't consciously directed) and you can have purpose without yet having earned its meaning (a direction you're still practicing into). The ideal is both — a life that feels worth living in the present and worth having lived in retrospect.

Life purpose is the quiet architecture underneath your choices — the through-line that gives shape and direction to the otherwise random events of a life. It's your particular blend of values, interests, skills, and lived experience, all pointing toward a direction that feels worth walking. When it's clear, it functions as an internal compass: helping you choose between paths, weather setbacks, and keep moving when the terrain turns difficult.

Purpose is not the cinematic 'calling' that descends in a single moment of clarity. More often it's a moving target — something that shifts as you do. In some seasons it arrives as a sharp point. In others it's a faint signal you track by trial and error. The mistake is waiting for certainty before taking the first step. Certainty about purpose is usually arrived at from the other direction: you move, you notice what feels alive and what doesn't, and you adjust. Purpose is practiced into existence, not received.

From a neurological perspective, purpose engages both brain systems in complementary ways. System 1 craves a purpose-shaped narrative — the primitive circuitry that asks 'am I doing something that matters to the group' is calmed by a felt sense of direction and contribution. System 2 thrives on purpose because it provides a framework for decision-making: without it, every choice requires fresh deliberation; with it, choices filter naturally through the question 'does this move me toward or away from what matters?'

Purpose tends to live at the intersection of three things:

1. What you care about deeply (the values that, when compromised, make you feel off-course)
2. What you're naturally drawn to or skilled at (the capacities that feel like second nature)
3. What the world needs that you can actually provide (the contribution that creates impact beyond yourself).

None of these three alone is sufficient. All three together describe a direction worth walking.

Why Purpose Is a Neurological Need, Not a Luxury

Purpose is not a reward you collect after the practical problems are solved. It is one of the practical problems. A life organized around borrowed goals, external benchmarks, and other people's definitions of success is not a stable life — it is a life that will eventually produce the question Paul was asking at midnight in an empty office: Is this it?

Neuroscience offers a specific answer to why. When behavior aligns with values, reward circuitry activates differently than it does when behavior is driven by external obligation. Dopamine release is steadier, more sustained, and more intrinsically motivated.[36] The motivational system designed to make you pursue things becomes an ally rather than an obstacle. Without values alignment, motivation becomes a finite resource you have to manufacture. With it, motivation becomes deeper and renewable.

The Cost of Neglect

- Aimlessness and distraction: Without a values-based filter, attention migrates toward whatever is most immediately stimulating rather than most genuinely important.

- Empty achievement: Goals reached without purpose alignment produce a specific kind of flatness — the 'is this it?' of Paul's Monday morning — that more achievement doesn't resolve.

- Fragile motivation: Purpose-free motivation is always borrowed from external sources. When the external rewards stop or feel insufficient, the motivation collapses with them.

- Identity confusion: Without a sense of direction, it becomes difficult to know who you are or make choices that feel authentically yours rather than inherited from others' expectations.

- Increased mental health vulnerability: Particularly at life transitions — retirement, loss, career shifts, relationship endings — where the external structures that provided a sense of purpose dissolve.

The Payoff of a Purpose-Oriented Life

- Resilient motivation: Values-driven action generates its own fuel. Setbacks are reframed as part of the direction of travel rather than evidence that the journey is wrong.

- Easier decisions: When you have a compass, choices filter naturally. You don't need to deliberate endlessly — you need to ask one question: does this move me toward or away from what matters?

- Psychological coherence: A life organized around values feels like yours — not arbitrary, not inherited, not performed for an audience. That coherence is itself a buffer against depression and anxiety.

- Sustainable fulfillment: Not the spike of achievement-based dopamine that fades, but the steady background hum of a life that feels worth living while you're living it.
- Contribution beyond self: Purpose that involves others creates meaning that persists beyond individual achievement — the relationships built, the people helped, the work that outlasts the effort.

Purpose and Long-Term Mental Health

The relationship between purpose and mental health has been studied more rigorously than most wellness writing suggests — and the findings are more specific and more powerful than the general claim that 'meaning is good for you.'

Viktor Frankl's logotherapy, developed through his observations in Nazi concentration camps and formalized in his book Man's Search for Meaning, established that the capacity to find or construct meaning in suffering was the primary variable differentiating those who survived psychologically intact from those who didn't.[35] This is not a soft finding. It's one of the most robust observations in the history of psychological trauma research: meaning functions as a buffer against the most extreme forms of human suffering, not by eliminating the suffering but by contextualizing it within a narrative that makes it bearable.

From a neurobiological standpoint, purpose-aligned behavior activates the prefrontal cortex's executive function in ways that externally-motivated behavior does not. When you're acting in service of something you genuinely care about, System 2 has a stable reference point — a north star that reduces the cognitive load of decision-making and provides a framework for evaluating experience. This is why purpose acts as a resilience resource: it doesn't prevent difficulty, but it changes how difficulty is processed. A setback in a purposeful life is information. A setback in a purposeless life is perceived as evidence of failure.

For depression specifically, purpose deficit and depression interact in a vicious loop: depression reduces the motivation and energy required to pursue purpose-aligned activities; the absence of purpose-aligned activity removes one of the most reliable sources of intrinsic dopamine; reduced intrinsic reward deepens depression. The loop tightens. The intervention — as Paul's story demonstrates — is not to solve the question of purpose before taking action. It is to take one small purpose-adjacent action and let the neurochemical signal from that action begin to open the loop.

For PTSD, meaning-making is a recognized component of evidence-based treatment[37] — specifically the capacity to integrate traumatic experience into a life narrative that is coherent and forward-directed rather than frozen at the point of injury. Purpose doesn't erase trauma. It provides the narrative context within which trauma becomes part of a story rather than the end of one.

Purpose is not the solution to mental health challenges. It is the orientation that makes recovery feel worth pursuing and ultimately effective.

How to Build a Practice of Purpose

Purpose is harder to operationalize than sleep or nutrition because it doesn't have a discrete behavior you can point to. You can't schedule "making meaning on Tuesdays at 10". What you can do is build the conditions — the reflective practices, the values-aligned actions, the environmental cues — that make purpose more likely to emerge and more likely to be recognized when it does.

The Four Drivers work here not by manufacturing purpose but by reducing the noise that drowns it out and increasing the signal from behaviors that are already, quietly, purpose-adjacent. Pay attention to what gives you energy. Do more of it deliberately. Let the pattern reveal itself.

Start Small

You don't need to know your purpose to take a purpose-adjacent action. You need to take enough purpose-adjacent actions to start recognizing what your purpose might be. Start with one. Let the signals accumulate.

- Spend two minutes journaling each morning on one question: what gave me genuine energy yesterday? Not productive energy — aliveness energy. Your brain learns from patterns. Track the pattern.

- Identify one values-aligned action to take this week — not a life overhaul, just one specific action. Help someone. Learn something. Make something. Do it and notice how it feels two hours later.

- Clarify one core value before attempting to map your entire purpose. What is the one thing, if consistently violated, that makes you feel most off-course? Start there.

Shape Your Environment

Purpose erodes in noisy environments, not because the noise is harmful but because it fills the attentional space where values-reflection could happen. Design your environment to keep your compass visible.

- Keep a written list of your core values somewhere you encounter daily — your desk, your bathroom mirror, your phone's lock screen. Not as inspiration, but as orientation. What you see regularly, you act toward.

- Place a card in your wallet or on your desk with your top three priorities for this season of your life. When you face a decision, the card is already there. You don't need to reconstruct your values under pressure.

- Create a brief personal life-vision statement — one sentence, not a paragraph — and keep it somewhere you see it daily. Not a manifesto. A compass heading. An intention. Revise it as you evolve.

The natural world is one of the most reliable environments for the kind of reflective clarity that purpose requires — and one of the most underused. This isn't mysticism. It's attentional economics. Purpose-reflection needs a specific quality of mental space: not fully occupied, not fully idle, but moving through something that occupies peripheral attention gently without demanding deliberate thought. Walking outdoors — especially in natural settings, along varied terrain, through parks or near water — creates exactly that quality of space. The mind is carried along by the movement and the mild stimulation of the environment, and in the freed-up cognitive space, the quieter signals become audible: what you've been avoiding, what actually matters, what you keep coming back to.

There is also a more direct mechanism. Dacher Keltner's research on awe — the state triggered by encountering something vast, complex, or incomprehensible — consistently shows that awe produces what he calls the "small self" response: a temporary reduction in self-referential thinking that paradoxically increases feelings of meaning, connection, and perspective. Natural environments are among the most reliable awe triggers available at low cost and no commute. A clear night sky. A forest path with old trees. The ocean at any hour. These are not aesthetic experiences. They are neurological events — brief disruptions of the default mode network's self-narrative that, with repetition, build a lasting orientation toward meaning beyond the personal. For people working on questions of purpose, regular exposure to natural scale is not optional background scenery. It is a direct input to the inquiry.

Link Habits

Purpose-reflection practices work best at transitions — the brief moments when attention is unscheduled. Attach them there and they become part of how you move between states rather than a separate task competing for time.

- After waking, before checking your phone, read one sentence from your values list or purpose statement. Not to be inspired — to orient. The day's first input shapes the day's default direction.
- Pair your morning walk, commute, or any regular solo movement with reflecting on one question: what would I do today if I were living fully from my values? You're moving anyway. Let the reflection catch a ride.
- Use the 5-4-3-2-1 countdown to act on a purpose-aligned opportunity before doubt or busyness generates a sufficient reason not to. The moment you notice something that aligns with what matters to you, count down and move.

Celebrate the Wins

Purpose-aligned actions often produce no external recognition. They may not impress anyone. They may not advance your career in obvious ways. The internal acknowledgment is therefore doing all of the reinforcement work — training your nervous system to recognize values-alignment as a reward in its own right, independent of outcome. Use it deliberately.

- After any values-aligned action — a conversation, a choice, a small act in the direction of what matters — take five seconds to acknowledge it. Not 'I'm living my purpose.' Just: 'That felt like me.' Your nervous system learns from that signal.

- Keep a daily log of purpose-driven actions — not to track your virtue, but to make the pattern visible. Purpose clarifies through accumulated evidence, not through a single moment of insight.
- Treat each aligned action as a practice rep for intentional living — not a test of whether you've found your purpose, but evidence that you're moving in a direction. Direction is what purpose actually is.

Your Action Steps

1. Start Small

Name one value-aligned action small enough to take this week without resolving the larger question of purpose:

- "The one value I most want to honor this week is ____________________. One specific action that would express that value is ____________________."
- "For the next seven days, I will spend ________ minutes each morning answering this question in writing: what gave me genuine, alive energy yesterday? I will do this immediately after ____________________."
- "The one context in which I most feel like myself — the activity, role, or situation where I feel most aligned — is ____________________. I will do or engage with that for ________ minutes this week."

2. Shape Your Environment

Design your environment to keep your compass visible before the noise fills the space:

- "I will write my __________________ (top three values, one-sentence mission, key priorities for this season) and place them in __________________ so I encounter them before I encounter anything else each morning."

- "I will remove or reduce __________________ (a specific source of purposeless noise or distraction) from my environment to create space for values-reflection that currently has no room."

- "I will create a brief personal mission statement — one sentence — by completing this phrase: I am here to __________________ so that __________________."

3. *Link Habits*

Attach purpose-reflection to transitions where attention is briefly unscheduled:

- "Immediately after __________________ (waking up, finishing my morning coffee, ending my workday), I will spend _______ minutes on __________________ (reading my values, journaling one reflection, noting what gave me energy today)."

- "I will pair my __________________ (morning walk, commute, workout) with reflecting on one question: __________________ (e.g., 'What would I do today if I were fully living my values?' 'What am I building with this week?')."

- "When a purpose-aligned opportunity appears — a conversation, a project, a small act in the direction of what matters — I will count __________________ and act before I finish, rather than waiting for a better time."

- "I will take _______ weekly 'purpose walk' — 20 to 30 minutes outside, alone, without a destination or agenda. No podcast, no call, no productivity. Just moving through the world and noticing what I notice. I will carry a small notebook to capture whatever surfaces. I am not looking for answers. I am creating the conditions in which the quieter signals can become audible."

4. Celebrate the Wins

Train your nervous system to recognize values-alignment as its own reward:

- "After any values-aligned action, I will take five seconds to say to myself: ____________________ (e.g., 'That felt like mine,' 'That's the direction,' 'I'm practicing this')."
- "I will keep a log of purpose-adjacent actions in ____________________ — not to measure my progress toward a fixed destination, but to make visible the direction I'm already moving in."
- "If I take one values-aligned action every day for ________ days, I will reward myself with ____________________."

My Purpose Commitment

Write it down. Name the value. Name the action. Keep it small enough that you'll actually do it this week.

New Behavior:
What values-aligned action will you take? What value does it serve?

The Setup:
How will you keep your compass visible in your daily environment?

The Trigger:
I will do this immediately before/after I:

The Celebration:
I will acknowledge this felt like mine by:

Becoming You

At first, meaning and purpose feel like a riddle you're supposed to solve before you're allowed to start living properly:

I should figure out my calling. I should find my passion. I should know what I'm here for.

'Should' doesn't survive busyness, doubt, or the daily evidence that you are not, in fact, living the life you're supposed to be living. Real purpose doesn't arrive as a lightning bolt of clarity. It grows through repeated, ordinary, almost invisible choices. Saying yes to the thing that feels alive and no to the thing that feels performed. Spending one evening a week on something that actually matters to you. Taking one small action in the direction of a value you've been honoring only in the abstract. Each act is a data point. The pattern is the thread you want to keep pulling on.

At first System 2 does all the work — the journaling, the reflection, the deliberate experiments in values-aligned living. It feels effortful, uncertain, occasionally absurd. But the data accumulates. The pattern clarifies. Each small action lays down a slightly clearer signal about what is and isn't yours — until the question of purpose stops feeling like a problem to be solved and starts feeling like a direction already in progress.

System 2 passes the baton to System 1. And purpose stops being something you're searching for and starts being something you're simply doing.

You are no longer drifting, measuring your life against borrowed benchmarks, waiting for clarity to arrive before you start moving. Purpose ceases to be a question you're asking of life. It becomes the answer you are living.

Paul got there. Not through a career epiphany or a single moment of clarity. Through walking into a legal aid clinic on a Tuesday evening and asking if they needed help, repeated until it became the direction his life was already pointing.

So can you.

Being of Service

Skill #9: The Contribution Principle

"The best way to find yourself is to lose yourself in the service of others."
— Mahatma Gandhi

Melanie

Melanie used to think of service as something other people did — the people with more time, more energy, more margin in their lives. The retired couples who volunteered at food banks on Thursday mornings. The childless colleagues who stayed late to mentor interns. The saints. Between a demanding job, two teenage kids whose schedules operated like competing logistical operations, and the endless churn of ordinary life, she told herself she'd give back once things calmed down.

But things never calmed down. They just changed shape.

One Saturday, leaving the grocery store, she noticed an older man struggling with bags near the exit. He was maybe seventy-five, slight, his fingers white around the plastic handles, leaning slightly as if the weight was winning. She almost kept walking — she had a list of things waiting for her at home, a car that needed unloading, kids who needed feeding, laundry that had been sitting in the dryer since Thursday. But something made her pause. She turned back, introduced herself, and carried his bags to the bus stop two blocks away. It took three minutes. He thanked her with a smile that reached his eyes and stayed with her — not for an hour, not for an afternoon, but for days. She kept returning to it the way you return to a song you can't quite place.

The next week, without planning it, she found herself knocking on the door of a neighbor who lived alone — an older woman she'd waved at for three years without ever really seeing. Then she started noticing more: a colleague whose eyes were red at the edges by Thursday afternoon, a stranger outside the pharmacy squinting at a paper map, a friend whose social media had gone quiet in a way that felt different from busy. Small things. Quiet things. The kind of things that don't make it into anyone's highlight reel. Acts that began, almost imperceptibly, to stitch her days together differently — to give them a shape she hadn't known they were missing.

At first she had to remind herself: do one small thing for someone else today. A Post-it on the bathroom mirror. An alarm on her phone. But over time the reminders stopped being necessary. Helping became part of how she moved through the world — as automatic and unquestioned as the way she brushed her teeth before bed or checked that the back door was locked.

Melanie no longer thought of herself as someone who should be more giving. She had become, without fanfare or announcement, a person who served. What surprised her most wasn't the impact on others — it was what happened inside her. It hadn't required a personality transplant or a sudden surplus of spare time. It had required only a willingness to pause — to let the needs of the moment matter as much as the list in her head. The capacity had always been there, coiled and waiting. She'd just never given it permission to show up.

And the shift wasn't only about the people she helped. Her days had a different texture now — less like a series of tasks to be defeated, more like a fabric she was actively weaving. The grocery run, the school pickup, the work call — they were the same as before. But threaded between them now were these small moments of contact, of usefulness, of genuine human exchange. They didn't slow her down. If anything, they made everything else feel less heavy.

In helping others find their footing, she found she was standing more solidly in her own.

Being of Service Quiz

Before we get into specifics, take two minutes to answer these questions. Answer honestly so you get a sense of how this past week has actually been for you.

This past week, how satisfied were you with your level of contribution and service?

⓪ Very dissatisfied ① Dissatisfied ② Fairly satisfied ③ Very satisfied

How capable did you feel of supporting and helping others?

⓪ Very incapable ① Somewhat incapable ② Fairly capable ③ Very capable

How motivated did you feel to be of service to others?

⓪ Very unmotivated ① Somewhat unmotivated ② Fairly motivated ③ Very motivated

How much did your engagement with others contribute to your sense of connection and belonging?

⓪ Not at all ① A little ② Fairly significantly ③ Significantly

How often did you engage in activities that helped or supported others?

⓪ Never ① Occasionally ② Often ③ Every day

Your Score: __________ (Total: 0–15)

- If 0–5: Begin with one small, consistent act of service per week. Frequency before scale.
- If 6–10: Align your contribution with your specific strengths and values. Effective service is targeted, not just frequent.
- If 11–15: Deepen your impact and protect against depletion. Service without self-care is a debt with interest.

What Being of Service Actually Is

Being of service is the act of turning outward — using your time, attention, skills, or resources to make someone else's load lighter, without keeping a private ledger of what they owe you in return. It might be as brief as holding the door for someone, carrying groceries to a bus stop or as dedicating years of work to a cause that will outlive you. The form is almost irrelevant. What defines service is the direction of the energy: away from yourself, toward another.

From an evolutionary standpoint, service wasn't charity. It was the operating principle of group survival. In small human bands, your survival was inseparable from everyone else's. You shared the meat because tomorrow you might be the one who came back empty-handed. You tended the injured because sooner or later you'd be the one limping. Reciprocity wasn't a virtue — it was the sustenance that kept everyone alive.

Your brain still runs that code. Acts of service activate the same reward pathways that once reinforced group cohesion: dopamine fires the 'this is good, do it again' signal; oxytocin releases the 'you're safe with these people' signal.[38] The neuroscience of altruism is not idealistic. It's ancient and self-interested in the deepest sense — a nervous system rewarding you for doing the thing that kept your ancestors alive.

Service exists in multiple forms, each engaging different capacities:

- Direct help — the physical and practical: carrying bags, giving a ride, fixing what's broken.
- Emotional support — the relational: listening without interrupting, staying steady through someone else's storm, offering presence when presence is what's needed.
- Skill sharing — the generative: teaching, mentoring, solving a problem that someone else can't crack alone.

- Stewardship of shared spaces — trail maintenance, community gardening, park cleanup, urban tree planting — these acts engage the same prosocial reward circuitry as direct personal service, with the added dimension of contributing to something that will outlast the act itself.

All three activate the same underlying circuitry. The scale doesn't change the mechanism. Three minutes at a bus stop produces the same neurochemical signal as three years building a nonprofit. System 1 doesn't measure impact. It measures direction.

Why Service Is a Survival Strategy, Not a Virtue

Service is not sainthood. It's not something you earn the right to engage in once you've resolved your own struggles, accumulated enough resources, or become a better person. It is one of the oldest adaptive behaviors in the human repertoire — a behavior your nervous system is actively designed to reward, because for most of human history, mutual contribution was the difference between a group that thrived and one that didn't.

In the short term, acts of service produce immediate and measurable neurochemical effects. Mood lifts. Rumination interrupts. The narrow tunnel of self-focus widens. Social bonds that were thin become slightly less so. These aren't poetic descriptions — they're the downstream effects of dopamine and oxytocin release in response to prosocial behavior. Your brain is paying you for helping. It has been doing this for a hundred thousand years.

The Cost of Neglect

- Narrow self-focus: Without the outward pull of contribution, rumination fills the space. Isolation compounds.
- Transactional relationships: Without genuine service, interactions stay at the surface — useful but not nourishing.

- Emotional stagnation: The specific quality of satisfaction that comes from giving freely doesn't come from any other source.
- Loss of perspective: Personal problems feel outsized when there's no context of others' needs to locate them against.
- Meaning deficit: A life organized entirely around personal acquisition and comfort tends, over time, toward a particular kind of emptiness that more acquisition doesn't fix.

The Payoff of Consistent Service

- Elevated mood: Prosocial behavior activates reward pathways reliably — not as a side effect, but as a direct neurochemical return.
- Stronger community bonds: Reciprocity builds belonging. People who help are helped. The network becomes denser and more trustworthy.
- Durable meaning and purpose: The sense that your existence matters to others is one of the most robust predictors of psychological well-being across cultures and across the lifespan.
- Resilience in personal adversity: Paradoxically, helping others through difficulty is one of the most reliable ways to develop perspective on your own.
- Identity consolidation: You become, over time, someone who contributes — and that identity is more stable and more satisfying than any identity built on personal achievement alone.

Service and Long-Term Mental Health

The relationship between service and mental health is bidirectional, and the mechanisms are specific enough to be worth naming precisely.

Depression characteristically narrows perspective — the world contracts until you feel like the only actor on the stage, the only person whose suffering is real, the only problem worth attending to. This isn't a moral failure. It's a neurobiological feature of depressive episodes, driven partly by dysregulated default mode network activity — the brain's self-referential circuitry running at abnormally high amplitude.[39] Service interrupts this loop by externalizing attention. You cannot simultaneously be fully absorbed in someone else's need and fully absorbed in your own rumination. The networks compete. Service wins.

Anxiety traps energy in internal loops — the rehearsal of future threats, the replay of past failures, the anticipatory scanning for danger that never resolves because the threat is never concrete enough to address. Service externalizes that energy into action with a visible outcome. You carried the bags. The neighbor is not alone today. The task is done and the result is real. Anxiety has difficulty sustaining itself in the presence of completed, concrete, other-directed action.

For PTSD specifically, service offers something that may be the most counter-intuitive intervention in this book: it gradually rebuilds trust through the experience of being useful to another person in a safe context. Trauma often severs the felt sense of being connected to — and capable of contributing to — the human world. Small acts of service restore that connection incrementally, in doses small enough that the threat response doesn't activate before the reward does.

Here is the vicious loop that a service deficit creates: isolation increases self-focus. Increased self-focus amplifies rumination.

Rumination worsens mood. Worsened mood reduces motivation to engage with others. Reduced engagement increases isolation. The loop tightens. Service — even one unremarkable act per week — introduces a counter-force into that loop. Not enough to break it immediately. Enough to create a crack.

Meaning is not found in solitude. It is found in the space between 'me' and 'them'. Service is how you enter that space deliberately.

How to Build a Service Practice

Most people who want to be of more service aren't blocked by selfishness. They're blocked by the overhead of deciding — whether now is a good time, whether their help would be welcome, whether it's enough to matter. The Four Drivers reduce that overhead by building service into the architecture of the day before the decision-fatigue kicks in.

The goal isn't to become a different kind of person. It's to lower the threshold between noticing an opportunity and acting on it — until System 1 starts doing the noticing automatically and System 2 can spend its energy on the more complex forms of service that require it.

Start Small

Three minutes at a bus stop counts. Your nervous system doesn't measure the scale of the act. It measures the direction. Start with something so small it would embarrass you to mention it — and notice what it does to your day.

- Commit to one small act of help per week. Not per day — per week. One. Carrying groceries, holding a door, sending a message to check in. Let the bar be genuinely low until the behavior is automatic.

- Give one genuine, specific compliment each day. Not flattery — something you actually noticed. 'You handled that meeting well.' 'That helped me.' Real observation, freely given.

- Choose one service skill to practice before trying to master them all. Active listening. Staying present without offering solutions. Showing up consistently. One skill, practiced with intention.

Shape Your Environment

Most missed opportunities to serve aren't failures of generosity. They're failures of attention. Design your environment to redirect attention outward before the moment passes.

- Keep a visible list of three to five people or situations where you could be of help — a family member, a friend, a neighbor, a colleague, a community need you've been meaning to address. What you can see, you act on.

- Place a prompt somewhere you'll encounter it daily — a question on your fridge, a note in your phone. 'Who could use something from me today?' Not as guilt, but as orientation.

- Sign up for one recurring volunteer commitment so the decision is already made and in your calendar. Consistency of environment is the fastest route to consistency of behavior.

Link Habits

Service behaviors are among the first to be displaced when the day gets demanding. Attach them to something that already runs automatically and they stop competing for schedule space.

- After finishing lunch — every day, not when you remember — send one message offering help, checking in, or expressing appreciation to someone. One message. Lunch is already automatic. Let the message catch a ride.

- Pair errand days or workout days with one act of service — dropping off donations, checking in on a neighbor, delivering something to someone who needs it. You're already moving through the world. Let it brush against someone else's life.

- Use the 5-4-3-2-1 countdown to act on an opportunity to help before hesitation generates a sufficient reason not to. The moment you notice someone who could use something, count down. Move before you finish. The hesitation loop can't complete if you're already in motion.

Celebrate the Wins

Acknowledging your acts of service isn't self-congratulation. It's the dopaminergic signal that tells your brain this behavior is worth repeating — which means more people get helped. The reinforcement is in service of the service.

- After any act of contribution — however small — take five seconds to acknowledge it internally. Not 'I'm a good person.' Just: 'I did that. That happened.' The circuit strengthens either way.

- Keep a brief service log — not to track your virtue, but to make your contribution visible to yourself. Over time, the log becomes evidence that you are, in fact, the kind of person who shows up for others.

- Treat each act of service as a practice rep for the skills of empathy, resourcefulness, and presence — skills that get sharper with use and that make every subsequent act more effective.

Your Action Steps

1. Start Small

Choose one act so small your brain can't negotiate its way out of it:

- "The one act of service I will do this week, no matter what, is ____________________ (e.g., text one person to check in, hold the door and make eye contact, bring something to a neighbor)."

- "The person in my life who could most use a small act of support right now is ____________________. The specific thing I could do for them is ____________________."

- "One service skill I want to practice this month is ____________________ (e.g., listening without offering solutions, following through on small offers, noticing need before being asked). I will practice it with ____________________."

- "I will identify ________ act of environmental stewardship — picking up litter on my regular walk, watering a neglected plant in a shared space, contributing an hour to a community garden or trail cleanup event — and treat it as a legitimate form of service, as valid as any other in this chapter. I will do it once this week and notice what it produces."

2. Shape Your Environment

Design your environment to redirect attention outward before the opportunity passes:

- "I will keep a list of ____________________ people or situations where I could be helpful in ____________________ (my phone notes, on my fridge, in my planner) so I see it regularly."

- "I will place a daily prompt — __________________ (a question, a word, a reminder) — in __________________ (my bathroom mirror, my phone lock screen, my desk) to orient me toward contribution each morning."

- "I will sign up for __________________ (a recurring volunteer commitment, a regular check-in with someone, a community activity) that happens on __________________ so the decision is already made."

3. Link Habits

Attach service to something that already runs automatically:

- "Immediately after __________________ (finishing lunch, completing my morning routine, ending my workday), I will __________________ (send one message of support, reach out to someone I've been meaning to contact, do one small act of help)."

- "I will pair my __________________ (weekly errands, Saturday morning, commute) with __________________ (dropping something off for a neighbor, a check-in call, a small act of contribution I've been putting off)."

- "When I notice an opportunity to help and feel the urge to hesitate, I will count __________________ and act before I finish. The hesitation is the signal to move, not to wait."

4. Celebrate the Wins

Reinforce the behavior so your nervous system encodes service as a reliable source of reward:

- "After any act of contribution, I will take five seconds to say to myself: __________________ (e.g., 'That mattered,' 'I showed up,' 'That's who I am')."

- "I will keep a brief log of my acts of service in ____________________ (a notebook, my phone, a habit tracker) — not to measure my virtue, but to make my contribution visible to myself."
- "If I complete one act of service every day for ________ days, I will reward myself with ____________________."

My Service Commitment

Write it down. Specific enough that you could describe it to someone else. Small enough that you'll actually do it.

New Behavior:
What, specifically, will you do? For whom?

The Setup:
How will you position yourself to notice and act on opportunities?

The Trigger:
I will do this immediately before/after I:

The Celebration:
I will acknowledge my contribution by:

Becoming You

At first, service feels like a noble intention:

I should volunteer more. I should check in on my neighbor. I should give back.

'Should' is no match for fatigue, busyness, or the ordinary gravitational pull of your own life. Real contribution doesn't emerge from grand gestures or annual charity drives. It grows through repeated, unremarkable acts. Holding the door. Sending the text. Staying an extra ten minutes. Carrying bags to a bus stop. Each act is small enough to be invisible and significant enough to change the texture of someone's day — including yours.

At first System 2 does all the work — the reminders, the deliberate choices, the moments of deciding to turn outward when turning inward would be easier. It feels effortful. But the repetitions accumulate. Each act lays down a slightly lower threshold for the next one, a slightly more automatic recognition of need, a slightly faster impulse to respond.

System 2 passes the baton to System 1. Helping stops being something you decide to do. It becomes something you simply notice yourself doing.

You are no longer someone who intends to give more. You are part of the living network of care and reciprocity that sustains human life. Not because you made a grand commitment to it, but because you showed up, quietly, enough times that it became indistinguishable from who you are.

Melanie got there. Not through volunteering or giving or any act large enough to name. Through carrying bags to a bus stop, three minutes at a time, until it became the kind of person she was.

So can you.

Joy, Play & Awe

Skill #10: The Art of Thriving

"Awe is the feeling of being in the presence of something vast that transcends your current understanding of the world."

— Dacher Keltner

"We don't stop playing because we grow old; we grow old because we stop playing."
— George Bernard Shaw

Bruno

Bruno was 42 and, by most external measures, doing fine. Stable IT job. A quiet apartment in a decent part of town. The kind of place that looked fine in photos and felt hollow in person. Enough streaming subscriptions to fill every evening with noise that passed for company. He wasn't unhappy, exactly. Unhappy would have been easier to diagnose, easier to fix. This was something more insidious — a slow, almost imperceptible draining of color from everything. Life had flattened into grayscale, and he'd been too busy to notice until the gray was all there was.

He couldn't remember the last time he'd belly-laughed. Not the polite chuckle he deployed in meetings, not the courtesy smile at a colleague's joke, but the kind of laughter that bends you in half and leaves you breathless. Couldn't remember the last time something had made him stop mid-stride and whisper wow. Even weekends, once a chance to exhale, had calcified into an endless loop of errands, meal prep, and the particular numbness of scrolling through other people's lives at 10pm on a Sunday.

One Saturday, in a state of malaise — the motivating force he'd been too proud to admit was running his decisions — he agreed to join a friend's pickup soccer game in the park. He hadn't played in twenty years. His cleats were somewhere in a closet. He borrowed a pair of sneakers and showed up expecting to feel old.

Within ten minutes he was sweaty, clumsy, and laughing harder than he had in months. Not at anything in particular. At everything. At the absurdity of his own stiff limbs, at the ball skidding wildly off his shin, at the mud that swallowed his left shoe completely on a poorly judged lunge. The game was thoroughly ordinary — a few friends, a patchy field, a scuffed ball that had lost most of its air. But for Bruno it cracked something open, like light through a door he'd forgotten existed. He remembered what it felt like to move for no reason. To play simply for the sake of playing, with no metric attached, no outcome to optimize, no version of himself to perform.

The following week he found himself lingering in the park longer than usual, watching kids chase each other with the kind of total abandon that adults spend years explaining away. He started bringing a sketchpad to the café on Sunday mornings — not to produce anything worth showing anyone, just to let his hand move across the page without agenda. One evening, mid-walk home from the train station, he looked up and felt small in the best possible way: a pink and gold sunset bleeding across the skyline, the kind he had passed a thousand times without ever actually seeing.

Over time, these moments stopped feeling like exceptions to his regular life and started feeling like the point of it. Bruno no longer thought of joy as something to hunt for on special occasions, some reward dispensed at the end of sufficient suffering. It began emerging naturally — quiet and unhurried, stitched into the fabric of ordinary days. He wasn't trying to be playful anymore. He was becoming someone for whom delight was simply a way of paying attention to the world that had been there all along.

Joy, Play & Awe Quiz

Before we get into specifics, take two minutes to answer these questions. Answer honestly so you get a sense of how this past week has actually been for you.

This past week, how satisfied were you with the amount of joy or awe you experienced?

⓪ Very dissatisfied ① Dissatisfied ② Fairly satisfied ③ Very satisfied

How many days did you engage in something playful — just because?

⓪ No days ① 1–2 days ② 3–4 days ③ Every day

How many days did you do something that made you laugh or smile genuinely?

⓪ No days ① 1–2 days ② 3–4 days ③ Every day

How many days did you learn something new or follow a thread of genuine curiosity?

⓪ No days ① 1–2 days ② 3–4 days ③ Every day

How many days did you feel genuinely curious about or interested in the people and world around you?

⓪ No days ① 1–2 days ② 3–4 days ③ Every day

Your Score: __________ (Total: 0–15)

- If 0–5: Start with one small daily joy ritual. Not a vacation. Not a transformation. One moment, deliberately noticed.
- If 6–10: Seek out more novelty, play, and beauty. Variety is the variable that keeps these states alive.
- If 11–15: Maintain joy, play, and awe as core life practices. These states erode under routine pressure. Protect them actively.

What Joy, Play & Awe Actually Are

Joy, play, and awe are three distinct neurological states that share a common property: they expand perception. Where chronic stress narrows attention to the immediate threat, these three states open it — widening the field of what you notice, what you consider possible, and who you feel connected to. They are not luxuries. They are the antidote to the tunnel vision that sustained stress produces.

Joy is a brief, system-wide lift — a moment when something in your environment lands just right and your nervous system registers it as unambiguously good. A laugh with a friend. Sunlight through leaves. The particular satisfaction of a sentence that comes out right. Joy is fleeting, but it leaves a neurochemical residue: dopamine and serotonin released in response to positive experience build a reserve that System 2 can draw on during harder moments. You are not just feeling good at the moment. You are stocking an emotional reservoir.

Play is an attitude, not an activity. It is self-directed, intrinsically motivated, and operating under low-stakes conditions where imagination runs higher and self-consciousness runs lower. In play, System 1 generates novel patterns freely, while System 2 occasionally refines or reframes without shutting the process down. The specific value of play is transfer: the flexibility and creativity rehearsed under low-stakes conditions is the same flexibility and creativity available under high-stakes ones. You are not wasting time when you play. You are training the cognitive architecture that handles difficulty.

Awe is the perceptual reset button. Standing before something vast — a night sky, a piece of music that opens something in your chest, the quiet face of a sleeping child — temporarily dissolves the default-mode network's self-referential chatter and produces what Dacher Keltner's research calls the 'small self' response: a brief shrinking of ego that paradoxically increases feelings of connection, meaning, and generosity. Neurobiologically, awe reduces inflammatory cytokines, lowers cortisol, and primes the nervous system for trust and openness. It is the moment when both brain systems — System 1's emotional immediacy and System 2's sense-making — agree to pay full attention at the same time. Those moments are rare. They are also, according to the research, the moments most associated with long-term psychological well-being.

All three states flourish in what psychologists call autotelic activities — things done purely for their own sake, without external goal or audience. Hiking without a step count. Sketching without posting. Cooking a new dish just to see what happens. These are not wasted hours. They are the conditions under which your nervous system remembers that not everything is transactional, not everything is a performance, and not everything has to produce a result whose value can be measured by money.

Why Joy, Play & Awe Are Non-Negotiable

Joy, play, and awe are not rewards you collect after the serious work is done. They are conditions that result from altered neurochemical states that your nervous system requires in regular doses to maintain cognitive flexibility, emotional resilience, and social connection that constitute psychological health. A life from which they are consistently absent is not a sustainable life.

The short-term costs of their absence are familiar to anyone who has spent too long in productivity mode without counterbalance: stress without release, thinking that narrows into tunnel vision, days that feel functionally complete but somehow hollow. These are not character flaws. They are the predictable results of a nervous system running on urgency without access to the perceptual reset that these three states provide.

The Cost of Neglect

- Perceptual narrowing: Sustained stress without joy or play produces tunnel vision — attention locked on threat, difficulty, and obligation, with no access to the wider field.

- Cortisol accumulation: Without regular release valves, stress hormones build. The nervous system stays in mild emergency mode indefinitely, producing the flatness and life in grayscale.

- Cognitive rigidity: Play and awe train flexibility. Without them, thinking becomes more rigid, problem-solving more rote, and creative capacity more constrained.

- Social thinning: Laughter and shared play are among the most reliable social bonding mechanisms available. Without them, relationships stay functional but not warm.

- Existential flatness: A life without moments of genuine delight and transcendence starts to feel like a series of tasks rather than an experience worth having.

The Payoff of Regular Joy, Play & Awe

- Perceptual expansion: These states widen what you notice, what you consider possible, and who you feel connected to — the opposite of the tunnel vision that chronic stress produces.

- Neurochemical restoration: Dopamine, serotonin, and oxytocin released through joy and awe build the reserves that support emotional regulation, social trust, and resilience.

- Cognitive flexibility: Play rehearses the adaptability that difficulty requires. The creativity and flexibility available in low-stakes play are the same capacities available in high-stakes situations.

- Deeper social connection: Laughter and shared awe are among the fastest routes to genuine intimacy. They bypass the performance layer that most social interaction requires.
- A life that feels worth living: Not the absence of difficulty, but the presence of enough delight that the difficulty is contextual rather than total. Living life in full color rather than grayscale.

Joy, Play & Awe and Long-Term Mental Health

The mental health case for joy, play, and awe is more specific and more robust than the general claim that 'positive experiences are good for you.' Each of the three states has a distinct and well-documented mechanism of action on the systems most implicated in depression, anxiety, and trauma.

Joy and positive affect, maintained consistently over time, are among the most reliable predictors of psychological resilience in longitudinal research. This is not because joy eliminates negative states but because it builds the emotional reserves that negative states draw down. Barbara Fredrickson's broaden-and-build theory establishes the mechanism: positive emotions broaden attention and cognitive flexibility in the moment, and over time build durable psychological resources[40] — stronger social bonds, greater problem-solving capacity, more adaptive coping — that persist long after the moment of joy has passed. You are not just feeling better when you experience joy. You are building infrastructure.

Play deprivation has measurable consequences. Stuart Brown's research on play — including studies of violent offenders and adults with chronic depression — found that play deprivation in childhood and adulthood is associated with rigidity, depression, and a reduced capacity for social connection.[41] Play is not developmental decoration. It is a biological requirement that doesn't expire at the end of childhood. Adults who maintain regular play behavior show lower baseline cortisol, greater cognitive flexibility, and more robust social bonds than those who don't.[41]

Awe, specifically, has the most surprising mental health research profile of the three states. Keltner's lab has demonstrated that awe experiences are associated with reduced levels of pro-inflammatory cytokines — the same markers elevated in depression, PTSD, and chronic stress.[42] A single awe experience measurably shifts the inflammatory profile of the nervous system. Regular and repeated exposure to awe — through nature, music, art, or human achievement — appears to sustain that reduction over time. Of these pathways, natural environments are the most reliably accessible for most people: they're free, they're available daily, and they don't require a gallery ticket, a concert hall, or a moment of someone else's extraordinary performance. What they require is attention — specifically, the deliberate decision to look at what is actually there rather than past it.

The research threshold for an awe response is lower than most people assume. You do not need Yosemite, a backflip on a motorcycle or a precise understanding of quantum physics. You simply need a cloud formation you've stopped long enough to actually see and appreciate. A spider web with dew on it. The particular quality of light at the end of winter that is different from any other kind of light. The fact that a single square meter of living soil contains more organisms than there are humans on Earth.[57] Natural environments are not depleted by attention the way human-made novelties are. They are inexhaustibly complex, and they reward looking in a way that screens and interiors don't, because the complexity is genuinely unresolvable. You're never 'done' looking at a forest. You can't fully understand a tide pool. That irreducible depth is precisely what produces the small-self response — the brief, restorative dissolution of the relentless self-centered narrative.

Here is the vicious loop that chronic deprivation of joy, play, and awe creates: chronic stress narrows perception and increases inflammatory load -> Narrowed perception makes it harder to notice opportunities for joy, play, or awe -> Reduced exposure to these states maintains the inflammatory load and perceptual narrowing -> The loop tightens.

Bruno's Saturday soccer game was not a distraction from his problem. It was the intervention.

Delight is not the opposite of seriousness. It is the physiological condition under which seriousness becomes useful and sustainable.

How to Build a Practice of Joy, Play & Awe

You cannot manufacture joy, play, or awe on demand. What you can do is stop scheduling them out — stop filling every available moment with productivity and obligation until delight has nowhere to land. The Four Drivers work here by creating conditions and removing friction rather than forcing outcomes. Lower the barrier to play. Put awe in your path. Let the states emerge rather than trying to produce them.

The shift Bruno made wasn't from joyless to joyful. It was from a life with no room for joy to a life with enough room that joy could find its way in. That's the whole intervention.

Start Small

The idea of 'embarrassingly small' is especially important in this chapter. Joy doesn't require a planned vacation. Play doesn't require an audience. Awe doesn't require a mountain. Two minutes outside noticing the light dancing in the tree tops. A doodle in the margin of your notebook. Looking up to notice the stars every evening. Start there. The nervous system doesn't measure the scale of the experience. It measures the quality of attention you bring to it.

- Spend two minutes outside each day noticing something visually novel — lights, colors, shadows, movement you normally walk past without registering. Not to achieve anything. Just notice. This is the foundational awe practice.

- Add one moment of play to your day — a doodle, a joke, a physical movement for no reason, a game. Not to produce anything. Just because. *Autotelic* means the behavior itself is the reward.

- Choose one autotelic activity to engage with this week — something you do purely for the experience of doing it. No goal. No audience. No result required. Note how it feels two hours later.

Shape Your Environment

Delight gets crowded out by the serious because the serious is always visible. Your email is always open. Your to-do list is always there. Joy, play, and awe require physical presence in your environment to compete — not as an obligation, but as a readily available alternative to the seriousness of life.

- Keep a musical instrument, sketchpad, novel, ball, or whatever your preferred play object is somewhere you can see it from your usual seat. The instrument in the case under the bed stays silent. The one leaning against the wall in the living room gets played.

- Place one small object of beauty or wonder in your primary workspace — a photo, a stone, a plant, a postcard. Not for decoration. As a micro-dose awe trigger. Something that occasionally catches your eye and briefly dissolves tunnel vision.

- Schedule one play break per week in your calendar — the same commitment level as a work meeting. Not because play requires scheduling, but because it requires protection from the things that will otherwise fill its place.

Link Habits

Joy, play, and awe produce no output and generate no external accountability. They are the first to be displaced when the day becomes demanding. Attach them to something already protected in your schedule and they become part of the structure rather than the casualty of it.

- After lunch — every day, not just when you feel like it — do something playful for five minutes. Not a task. Not a check-in. Something that makes you smile or moves your body for no reason. Let the lunch break be the anchor.

- Pair outdoor movement and walks with awe-adjacent routes or destinations — a park, a view, a street with interesting light. You're moving anyway. Let what you move through change what you notice.

- Use the 5-4-3-2-1 countdown to drop into a playful activity the moment the impulse arises, before self-consciousness or productivity guilt talks you out of it. The impulse is the signal. Take action before it passes.

Celebrate the Wins

Joy, play, and awe are already their own reward — the dopamine is built in. The celebration here is not about adding a reward that isn't there. It's about pausing long enough to let the reward register before the seriousness of life pulls your attention away. The moment passes quickly. You have to deliberately hold it for a few seconds longer than feels normal.

- After any moment of genuine joy, play, or awe — however brief — pause for five seconds and let it land. Don't immediately move to the next thing. Let your nervous system register that just happened. That was good. This deliberate pause is the difference between something being a mere 'happening' versus an experience that gets woven into the fabric of your being.

- Keep an awe and joy log — not a gratitude list, something more specific. What was interesting today? What made you laugh? What felt genuinely alive? The pattern that emerges over weeks is a map of your particular version of delight. Follow it.

- Treat each intentional moment of joy, play, or awe as a practice rep for the skill of noticing — because that's what it is. Bruno didn't find a different life. He developed the attentional habit of seeing the one he already had.

Your Action Steps

1. Start Small

Choose one act of noticing or playing so small it requires no preparation and no justification:

- "My one daily joy ritual, starting this week, is ____________________ (e.g., two minutes outside noticing the light, one genuine laugh, one moment of deliberate stillness). I will do it immediately after ____________________."

- "The autotelic activity I most want to reclaim — the thing I used to do just because I loved it — is ____________________. I will spend ________ minutes on it this week, with no goal and no audience."

- "The last time I felt genuinely awe-struck was ___________________. I will put myself in proximity to that kind of experience this week by ___________________."

- "I will choose ______ natural object — a cloud, a tree, a patch of lichen, a spider web, the sky at a specific time of day — and spend 90 seconds looking at it as if I've never seen anything like it. I will do this daily for one week and track what I notice."

2. Shape Your Environment

Put delight in your path before the serious fills the space:

- "I will place ___________________ (instrument, sketchpad, ball, novel, object of beauty) in ___________________ so it's visible from where I spend most of my time."

- "I will add one awe trigger to my primary workspace — ___________________ (a photo, a plant, a natural object, a piece of art) — placed where it is likely to catch my eye."

- "I will protect one ___________________ (weekly play break, monthly adventure, regular time in nature) by blocking it in my calendar as non-negotiable, the same way I block medical appointments."

- "I will identify one outdoor location within 10 minutes of where I live or work that has reliable access to natural beauty — and designate it as my weekly awe appointment. I will go there ______ times a week with no agenda and no device, for a minimum of _______ minutes."

3. Link Habits

Attach joy, play, and awe to something that is already baked into your schedule:

- "Immediately after __________________ (lunch, my morning walk, finishing my workday), I will spend _______ minutes on __________________ (something playful, a route with beauty, a moment of deliberate noticing)."
- "I will pair my __________________ (daily walk, commute, workout) with __________________ (an awe-adjacent route, a piece of music that moves me, five minutes of genuine play before or after)."
- "When I feel the impulse to play or notice something beautiful, I will count to ____ and act on it before productivity guilt talks me out of it."

4. Celebrate the Wins

Let the experience land before the next thing takes over:

- "After any moment of genuine joy, play, or awe, I will pause for _______ seconds and let it register before moving on. I will say to myself: _________________________ (e.g., 'That was real,' 'I notice that,' 'More of that')."
- "I will keep an awe and joy log in __________________ — not what I'm grateful for in the abstract, but specifically what stopped me, what made me laugh, what felt alive."
- "If I have one genuine moment of joy, play, or awe every day for _______ days, I will reward myself with __________________."

My Joy, Play & Awe Commitment

Write it down. Name the condition. Name the act. Keep it small enough to be genuinely playful rather than another obligation.

New Behavior:
What will you do, just because? (No goal. No result required.)

The Setup:
How will you put delight in your path before the serious fills the space?

The Trigger:
I will do this immediately before/after I:

The Celebration:
I will pause and let it land by:

Becoming You

At first, joy feels like a luxury you'll get to when things settle down:

I should laugh more. I should take a break. I should find time for fun.

'Should' doesn't survive the serious. The deadlines are always real, the obligations are always there, and the part of you that was taught to equate value with productivity will always find a reason to defer delight to later. Real joy doesn't come from clearing enough space or earning enough rest. It grows through repeated, unremarkable, almost embarrassingly small acts. Two minutes noticing the light. A doodle that no one sees. Looking up at a sky you've passed under a thousand times and finally letting it be vast.

Each act is a practice rep for the skill of noticing. And noticing, practiced consistently, becomes a way of moving through the world — not a separate activity you add to your schedule but the quality of attention you bring to the schedule you already have.

At first System 2 does all the work — the reminders, the scheduled play breaks, the deliberate choices to look up rather than scroll down. It feels effortful and slightly awkward, the way any new attentional habit does. But the reps accumulate. Each small moment of delight lays down a slightly lower threshold for the next one, a slightly more automatic noticing of what's already there.

System 2 passes the baton to System 1. And joy stops being something you plan for and becomes something you simply notice happening.

You are no longer waiting for the right circumstances, the right vacation, the right grand experience to deliver the aliveness you've been deferring. You are becoming someone for whom delight is a mode of paying attention — available in a muddy soccer field, a café sketchpad, a pink and gold sky. Not a category of special experience.

A quality of ordinary presence. Delight ceases to be a rare visitor. It becomes part of who you are.

Bruno got there. Not through a transformed life. Through a Saturday soccer game and a sketchpad and the habit of looking up, repeated until delight became the way he moved through the life he already had.

So can you.

Conclusion

Where to Start, and Why It Matters That You Do

"I never see what has been done; I only see what remains to be done.."

— Marie Curie

"You are entitled to the action, but never to its fruits."

— Bhagavad Gita

Where to Start

You have just read ten chapters. Ten non-negotiables, ten quizzes, ten commitment pages, ten sets of action steps. If you're feeling slightly overwhelmed by the scope of what you've just been asked to consider — that's appropriate. You've just surveyed the entire architecture of your well-being.

It makes sense that you might find yourself asking, now what? Where do I actually start?

The answer is 'not everywhere.' Trying to improve all ten simultaneously is the fastest route to improving none of them. Behavior change research is unambiguous on this point: the more changes you attempt at once, the higher the cognitive load, the sooner the motivation collapses, and the more likely you are to revert to baseline by the third week.

You start with one. Then another. Then another after that. And you choose which one through a simple diagnostic, not a gut feeling.

The Three-Tier Model

The ten non-negotiables are not equal in their urgency or their sequencing. They form a hierarchy — one that mirrors the architecture of a house being built from the ground up. You've seen this metaphor in the introduction. Now it becomes practical. It must be practical in order for changes to stick.

Tier 1 — The Foundation

Sleep · Movement · Nutrition & Hydration

These are the biological prerequisites. They operate at the level of the nervous system, the immune system, the endocrine system - biological foundation of your organism. Every other non-negotiable runs on top of them. If your sleep is chronically poor, your emotional regulation is impaired before the day has started. If you are consistently under-nourished or sedentary, your cognitive capacity and mood regulation are compromised in ways that make progress in the other seven domains harder and slower.

The construction rule is simple: you cannot build on a foundation that isn't solid. If you scored 0–5 on any of the three Tier 1 quizzes, start there. Not because the other non-negotiables don't matter — they do — but because improving them will be harder and less durable until your biological floor is more stable.

Tier 2 — The Structure

Self-Care · Physical Environment · Life Administration

These are the structural systems that create the conditions for stability. Self-care keeps your window of tolerance open. Your physical environment shapes behavior below the level of conscious decisions. Life administration removes the chronic low-level cortisol load of unresolved obligations. Together, they create the organized, regulated context within which the Tier 3 non-negotiables can take root.

If your Tier 1 scores are reasonable but your Tier 2 scores are low, this is likely where your highest leverage lies. A person who sleeps adequately but lives in chronic administrative chaos and environmental disorder is still running with a significant drag on their system.

Tier 3 — Thriving

**Community & Belonging · Being of Service ·
Meaning & Purpose · Joy, Play & Awe**

These are the non-negotiables that make life feel worth living rather than merely functional. Thriving requires the foundation and structure to be reasonably stable before they can be built and sustained. You can have a flash of connection, a moment of purpose, a day of joy — but consistent, durable thriving in these domains is much harder to maintain if you're struggling with foundational and structural issues (your sleep is chronically disrupted and your kitchen is underwater).

If your Tier 1 and Tier 2 scores are healthy but your Tier 3 scores are low — you feel stable but empty, functional but not fully alive — this is where your attention belongs.

Finding Your Starting Point

Go back to the quiz in each chapter and write your score in the table below. Then identify where the lowest scores cluster. That cluster is your starting point.

My Ten Non-Negotiables Scores

Non-Negotiable	Tier	My Score
Sleep	1	
Movement	1	
Nutrition & Hydration	1	
Self-Care	2	
Physical Environment	2	
Life Administration	2	
Community & Belonging	3	
Meaning & Purpose	3	
Being of Service	3	
Joy, Play & Awe	3	

Look at where your lowest scores cluster. That's where to start. If any of your Tier 1 scores are low, then begin there regardless of what the Tier 3 scores say. If your foundation is shaky, building higher will only make the instability more visible.

The Golden Rule of Construction

When you feel stuck at a higher tier — when you can't find your purpose, can't build community, can't access joy — the solution is almost always found one tier down. A person who can't seem to stay socially connected may first need better sleep. A person who can't find meaning may first need to clear the administrative backlog that has been draining their cognitive bandwidth for months.

Fix the wall before you hang the painting. Fix the floor before you fix the wall. The sequence matters.

Your Starting Contract

Before you close this book, write down three things. Not ten. Just three.

The non-negotiable I will focus on first:

(choose the one with the lowest score, or the one causing the most friction)

The one specific behavior I am committing to this week:

The existing habit I will attach it to:

That's enough.

One non-negotiable. One behavior. One anchor. Do that until it's no longer an effortful decision. Then come back and pick the next one.

Why This Work Matters

What I've learned after nearly a decade in clinical medicine, most of it working with people in serious psychological distress is that the patients who recover most fully — not just stabilize, not just manage, but genuinely recover and build lives that feel worth living — are almost never the ones with the best medication regimens or the most sophisticated therapy protocols or the most number of Ketamine treatments. They are the ones who are able to build their foundation, then create structure and finally add their own decor of love, compassion and connection.

They start sleeping more consistently. They move their bodies, even a little. They clear the pile of unopened mail. They text one person instead of isolating. They step outside in the morning. They make themselves a real meal. None of these acts are dramatic. None of them photograph well. None of them would make a compelling or dramatic social media post. But collectively, over weeks and months, they construct something that no clinical intervention alone can build: a life with enough structure, enough biology, enough connection, and enough meaning that the mind has somewhere stable to land.

On a daily basis I bear witness to how Ketamine can open neurological windows that years of prior treatment hadn't touched. I have watched those windows close again, quickly, in patients who returned to the same depleted conditions that had generated the crisis in the first place. And I have also watched those windows stay open — and widen — in patients who used them to build something different. Not something perfect. But something real and sustainable nonetheless.

The ten non-negotiables are not a theory of everything. They will not resolve trauma, eliminate genetic vulnerability, or substitute for clinical treatment when clinical treatment is what's needed. What they will do — what I have watched them do, repeatedly, in people who did not believe they were capable of it — is create the conditions under which recovery becomes possible and thriving becomes imaginable.

That is not a small thing. For many people, it is everything.

On the Question of Perfection

You will not do all ten of these well. Not this month, probably not this year. Some of them will feel impossible given your current circumstances. Some of them will click into place quickly and surprise you. Some you will work on for years.

That is not failure. That is the nature of skills. Beth didn't fix her sleep in a week. Marcus didn't reclaim his body in a month. Jennifer didn't clear her inbox that afternoon.

They made one small change, noticed it mattered, and made another. The identity shift — the moment when they stopped trying to do something and became someone who simply did it — came later, and quietly, and without announcement.

It will come for you the same way. Not through a decision to change, but through the accumulation of small decisions, each one unremarkable on its own, each one laying down a thin layer of new neural infrastructure until the person you're trying to become is simply the person you are.

There are no shortcuts. But there is a direction. And now you have a map.

Ten People. Ten First Steps.

Before you go, a brief return to the people you met in these pages — because their stories are not separate from yours. They are a preview of what becomes possible when you do the work.

- Beth stopped scrolling in bed, slept deeper, and became a rested mother who could finally engage.
- Marcus walked around the block in old running shoes until movement stopped being penance and became practice.
- Mark poured a glass of water before his morning coffee and started, quietly, to trust his own body again.
- Lusia sent one text on a Sunday morning after coffee until she was no longer pressing her face against the glass.
- Arthur took one slow breath before reaching for his phone and, over time, became a man who steered his days instead of surviving them.
- Melanie opened doors for strangers and found herself re-rooted in her own life.
- Daniel moved a pair of shoes and opened the blinds until a thousand tiny pebbles had been removed from his shoes.
- Jennifer opened one envelope with a friend beside her and rebuilt, slowly, the capacity to trust herself.
- Paul walked into a legal aid clinic on a Tuesday evening and practiced his way into a life that felt alive.

- Bruno played a muddy soccer game and rediscovered that delight was not a destination but a way of paying attention.

None of them did anything extraordinary. All of them did something real. That distinction is the whole point of this book.

There are no shortcuts.

There is only the next small act — unglamorous, unremarkable, and yet entirely profound and completely sufficient.

Try it.

Appendix

A Reference Guide to Tools, Techniques, and Key Concepts

The action steps in this book draw on a consistent set of behavioral science methods, and the chapters reference a range of scientific concepts that are explained once and then applied throughout. This appendix collects all of them in one place, alphabetically, so you can look up what you need without hunting through chapters.

Each entry notes where the term appears in the book. Some entries are tools — things you do. Others are concepts — things that explain why the tools work. Most are both.

ACE Score (Adverse Childhood Experiences)

Where you'll find it: Introduction

The ACE questionnaire was developed in 1998 by researchers at Kaiser Permanente and the Centers for Disease Control. It consists of ten yes/no questions covering childhood exposure to abuse, neglect, and household dysfunction — including physical, emotional, and sexual abuse; household substance abuse; parental mental illness; domestic violence; and parental incarceration. Your score is the number of yes answers.

An ACE score of four or more is clinically significant. Research on over 17,000 participants found that a score of four or higher correlates with a 500 percent increase in risk of depression, a 1,200 percent increase in the risk of attempted suicide, and substantially elevated risk of cardiovascular disease, obesity, and other chronic health conditions. Roughly half the patients who come through CIT Clinics have scores of four or higher.

The purpose of knowing your score is not to locate blame or to calcify a narrative of damage. It is to understand that many of the behavioral patterns, emotional reactivity, and self-regulatory struggles covered in this book have origins that predate any adult decision you made. The brain was hyperplastic during those early years. Whatever happened — or didn't happen — got wired in. That wiring can be updated. It requires more repetition than pathways established later in life, and more patience. But the mechanism is identical: neurons that fire together, wire together.

The ten ACE questions:

1. Before your 18th birthday, did a parent or other adult in the household often swear at you, insult you, put you down, or humiliate you? Or act in a way that made you afraid you might be physically hurt? (emotional abuse)
2. Did a parent or other adult in the household often push, grab, slap, or throw something at you? Or ever hit you so hard that you had marks or were injured? (physical abuse)
3. Did an adult or person at least five years older than you ever touch or fondle you or have you touch their body in a sexual way? Or try to or actually have oral, anal, or vaginal sex with you? (sexual abuse)
4. Did you often feel that no one in your family loved you or thought you were important or special? Or that your family didn't look out for each other, feel close to each other, or support each other? (emotional neglect)
5. Did you often feel that you didn't have enough to eat, had to wear dirty clothes, and had no one to protect you? Or that your parents were too drunk or high to take care of you or take you to the doctor if you needed it? (physical neglect)
6. Were your parents ever separated or divorced? (household separation)

7. Was your mother or stepmother often pushed, grabbed, slapped, or had something thrown at her? Or sometimes or often kicked, bitten, hit with a fist, or hit with something hard? Or ever repeatedly hit over at least a few minutes or threatened with a gun or knife? (domestic violence)
8. Did you live with anyone who was a problem drinker or alcoholic, or who used street drugs? (substance abuse in household)
9. Was a household member depressed or mentally ill, or did a household member attempt suicide? (mental illness in household)
10. Did a household member go to prison? (incarceration in household)

Score one point for each yes. A score of zero doesn't mean your childhood was without difficulty — it means the specific adversities measured by this tool were not part of your experience. A score of four or more is the threshold associated with significant long-term health effects.

Allostatic Load

Where you'll find it: Physical Environment

Allostatic load is the cumulative biological cost of chronic stress — the wear and tear that accumulates across the body's regulatory systems when the stress response is activated repeatedly or persistently without adequate recovery.

The concept was developed by neuroscientists Bruce McEwen and Eliot Stellar in the early 1990s as a more precise alternative to the generic concept of "stress." Allostasis refers to the body's ability to maintain stability through change — the hormonal, cardiovascular, immune, and neural adjustments the body makes in response to demands. Allostatic load refers to the cost of those adjustments over time.

In the short term, allostatic responses are adaptive. Cortisol mobilizes energy for a demanding situation. Elevated blood pressure delivers more oxygen to working muscles. The immune system primes for potential injury. The problem is that these systems were designed for acute stressors — the threat that appears, demands a response, and resolves. In modern life, many stressors are chronic, low-level, and unresolvable: financial pressure, relationship conflict, a disordered physical environment, an administrative backlog, chronic sleep loss. The allostatic response stays active. The load accumulates.

High allostatic load is associated with accelerated aging of the cardiovascular, immune, and neuroendocrine systems; increased risk of depression, anxiety, and PTSD; impaired memory and executive function; and shortened lifespan. It is one of the mechanisms through which chronic psychological stress becomes physical illness.

Every chapter in this book addresses allostatic load, whether it names it or not. Sleep, movement, nutrition, self-care, environmental order, social connection — each of these is, among other things, an allostatic load management strategy. The goal is not the absence of stress. It is the presence of enough resilience and recovery that the load doesn't compound into damage.

Attention Restoration Theory

Where you'll find it: Self-Care , Physical Environment

Attention Restoration Theory was developed by environmental psychologists Rachel and Stephen Kaplan at the University of Michigan in the 1980s and 1990s. It proposes that there are two qualitatively different types of attention — directed attention and involuntary attention — and that they have fundamentally different resource requirements.

Directed attention is effortful and finite. It is what you use to write, read critically, plan, make decisions, manage complex social situations, and resist impulses. Extended use of directed attention depletes it — a phenomenon consistent with what the Life Administration chapter calls decision fatigue. The research term for this depletion is directed attention fatigue, and its symptoms are familiar: difficulty concentrating, irritability, impulsivity, reduced capacity for nuanced judgment, and the experience of being "done" cognitively long before the day is over.

Involuntary attention is effortless and restorative. It is drawn in automatically by stimuli that are inherently interesting without being demanding — a fire, moving water, clouds, birdsong, an irregular skyline of trees. Natural environments are the most reliable sources of involuntary attention triggers that humans have reliable access to, because they evolved in those environments and their sensory systems are tuned to them.

The practical implication: time in natural environments allows directed attention to recover while involuntary attention is gently and pleasurably occupied. This is why a twenty-minute walk in a park often produces more cognitive restoration than twenty minutes of rest indoors. Indoors rest tends to involve low-level directed attention — the mind drifts to problems, to-do lists, interpersonal concerns. Nature engages the involuntary system and gives the directed system something it rarely gets: an actual break.

For self-care, this means natural environments are one of the few restoration contexts that are both free and reliably effective. For environmental design, it means that access to natural light, views of trees or sky, and outdoor spaces should be treated as functional inputs to cognitive performance, not aesthetic luxuries.

BDNF (Brain-Derived Neurotrophic Factor)

Where you'll find it: Movement, Sleep, Nutrition & Hydration.

BDNF is a protein produced in the brain and nervous system that supports the survival of existing neurons, promotes the growth of new synaptic connections, and increases the plasticity of neural pathways — the ease with which they can be modified through experience and repetition. The neuroscientist and author John Ratey, drawing on decades of exercise research, calls it "Miracle-Gro for the brain." This is a useful metaphor: BDNF is to neural growth what fertilizer is to plant growth. It doesn't create the plant, but it creates the conditions under which growth is possible and efficient.

BDNF levels are elevated by: cardiovascular exercise, strength training, quality sleep, caloric restriction, certain dietary components (particularly omega-3 fatty acids), and — based on emerging research — exposure to natural environments. BDNF levels are suppressed by: chronic stress, sleep deprivation, social isolation, a sedentary lifestyle, and chronic inflammation.

Depression is associated with chronically reduced BDNF, particularly in the hippocampus (the brain region most associated with memory and emotional regulation) and the prefrontal cortex. Antidepressants produce some of their effects by upregulating BDNF. Ketamine produces a rapid and substantial BDNF surge, which is part of the mechanism behind its rapid antidepressant effects and the neuroplasticity window it creates.

For our purposes, BDNF is the molecular currency of the kind of change this book is about. Every behavior that increases BDNF — exercise, adequate sleep, quality nutrition, time in nature — is simultaneously making neuroplastic change easier, faster, and more durable. The chapter on Movement gives the most detailed treatment, but the BDNF connection is present in nearly every non-negotiable.

Broaden-and-Build Theory

Where you'll find it: Joy, Play & Awe

Broaden-and-Build theory was developed by psychologist Barbara Fredrickson at the University of North Carolina and is one of the most influential frameworks in positive psychology research.

The core argument has two parts.

First, positive emotions broaden cognition in the moment: when you experience joy, curiosity, awe, love, or contentment, your attentional field expands, your thinking becomes more flexible and creative, and you are more open to novel information and perspectives. This is the opposite of what negative emotions do — fear and anger narrow attention to the immediate threat, which is adaptive in a crisis but constraining in ordinary life.

Second, this broadening builds durable psychological resources over time: stronger social bonds (because positive states make you more open and generous in interaction), greater cognitive flexibility (because the broader attentional field of positive states exposes you to more information and creative combinations), more robust coping strategies (because repeated positive experiences give you more material to draw on under pressure), and improved physical health (through measurable reductions in inflammatory markers).

The implication that matters most for this book: joy, play, and awe are not rewards you collect after the real work is done. They are an input to the system that makes the real work more possible and more durable. A life reliably punctuated by positive emotional experience is not a soft aspiration. It is a strategic investment in the cognitive and emotional resources that hard things require.

Decision Fatigue

Where you'll find it: Life Administration, Life Administration

Decision fatigue is the degradation of decision quality that occurs after a person has made a sustained series of decisions. It was identified through research by social psychologist Roy Baumeister and his colleagues, who proposed that self-regulatory capacity — including decision-making — draws on a limited cognitive resource that is depleted by use.

The most striking empirical demonstration comes from a study of Israeli parole board judges, published in 2011: the probability of a favorable parole ruling was roughly 65 percent at the start of a session and dropped close to zero by the end, recovering sharply after each food break. The content of the cases had no systematic relationship to the time of day. The judges' mental fatigue did. This is decision fatigue in a high-stakes, real-world context.

In daily life, decision fatigue manifests as: an increasing tendency to choose the default option (inertia), impulsive choices made to end the decision process, avoidance of decisions altogether, reduced tolerance for nuance or complexity in options, and deteriorating self-control in areas unrelated to the decisions being made (more likely to eat impulsively, react emotionally, or skip established habits late in a cognitively demanding day).

The management strategies distributed throughout the Life Administration chapter — batching similar decisions, establishing routines that remove repeated choices, doing important decisions early in the day, reducing the total number of decisions through systems — are all decision fatigue interventions. So is the brief outdoor walk described in the new nature insertion: micro-exposures to natural environments measurably restore directed attention capacity, which is the same resource decision fatigue depletes.

The Four Drivers of Behavior Change

Where you'll find it: Introduction, then applied throughout every chapter

The Four Drivers appear in every chapter's "How to Build Skills" section in the same sequence: Start Small, Shape Your Environment, Link Habits, Celebrate Wins. This entry is a quick reference for applying them to behaviors not covered in the ten chapters, or for troubleshooting why a habit isn't sticking.

Start Small works because System 1 treats large changes as threats and generates resistance. Small changes slip through. The goal is not an impressive performance. The goal is the first rep — because the first rep is the neural event that makes the second rep more likely. If a new behavior isn't happening, make it smaller until it's embarrassingly easy. Then make it automatic before you make it bigger.

Troubleshooting: Is this small enough to do on your worst day of the year?

Shape Your Environment works because your environment makes most of your decisions before you're consciously aware a decision is being made. Willpower is finite and gets tired. Environmental design doesn't. The goal is to make the right behavior the path of least resistance and the wrong behavior require deliberate effort.

Troubleshooting: What would your environment have to look like for this behavior to happen automatically?

Link Habits works because new behaviors need reliable cues, and existing behaviors are the most reliable cues available. You're not building a new pathway from scratch — you're attaching a new pathway to an existing one so it inherits its automaticity. The trigger must be specific, consistent, and immediately preceding the new behavior.

Troubleshooting: What already-automatic behavior could serve as the trigger for this one?

Celebrate Wins works because the moment immediately following a new behavior is the neurological window in which the habit circuit either strengthens or stalls. A genuine internal acknowledgment — "good," said and meant — fires the same dopaminergic signal as external praise. Skip it and you leave the most powerful reinforcement mechanism unused. The celebration must be immediate (within seconds) and genuine (performed celebration doesn't work).

Troubleshooting: Are you pausing long enough after the behavior for your nervous system to register it as a good outcome?

5-4-3-2-1 Countdown

Where you'll find it: Self-Care, Life Administration, Community & Belonging

The 5-4-3-2-1 countdown is not a motivational trick. It's a neurological interrupt.

When you feel the pull toward avoidance — the impulse to delay, scroll, retreat, or snap — what's actually happening is that System 1 is running a pattern it knows well. The longer you let the pattern run, the more momentum it builds. Within seconds, your nervous system has generated a compelling case for not doing the thing. The window closes.

The countdown interrupts that process before it can complete. Counting backward out loud — five, four, three, two, one — engages the prefrontal cortex just long enough to create a gap between the impulse and the action. You're not summoning willpower. You're creating a two-second pause in which a different choice becomes possible.

The key is to move — physically, literally — before you finish counting. Not after. Before. Once your body is in motion, System 1 updates its read of the situation: apparently we're doing this. The internal argument loses its audience.

You're not waiting to feel ready. You're acting your way into readiness. That sequence — action first, feeling second — is the opposite of how most people assume motivation works. It is, however, how it actually works.

Count. Move. The rest follows.

Habit Stacking

Where you'll find it: Movement, Sleep, Self-Care, Community & Belonging, Life Administration — the "Link Habits" section of every chapter

Habit stacking is the practice of attaching a new behavior to an existing one — using an already-automatic behavior as the trigger for a not-yet-automatic one.

The underlying logic is neurological. Every established habit in your life is a well-grooved neural pathway that your brain runs with minimal effort or deliberation because it has been practiced hundreds or thousands of times. System 1 owns it. When you attach a new behavior to an existing one, the new behavior inherits some of that automaticity. The existing habit fires; the new one catches a ride.

"After I brush my teeth, I will write one sentence in my journal" is not a clever life hack. It's the application of a specific principle about how the brain builds new pathways: new behaviors need cues, and existing behaviors are the most reliable cues available.

The critical design choice is sequence. The new behavior must follow the existing one immediately — not around the time that you brush your teeth, not after you've had a chance to settle in. Immediately after. The tighter the temporal coupling, the more reliably the trigger fires the new behavior.

Start by listing the behaviors that already run automatically in your life: making coffee, sitting down at your desk, finishing lunch, locking the front door. These are your attachment points. For each new behavior you're building, find the existing habit that most naturally precedes it, and write the implementation intention accordingly.

Identity-Based Framing

Where you'll find it: Every "Becoming You" section at the end of each chapter

Identity-based framing is the practice of describing a behavior in terms of the kind of person who does it, rather than in terms of the outcome the behavior is meant to produce.

"I'm trying to exercise more" is outcome-based. "I'm someone who moves every day" is identity-based. The difference is not motivational poetry. It is a functional difference in how System 1 processes the behavior.

System 1 runs on identity. It constantly cross-references your actions against an internal model of who you are, filtering for consistency. When your actions conflict with your identity, System 1 generates friction. When your actions align with your identity, System 1 executes them more smoothly, defends them against competing impulses, and rebuilds them faster after disruption.

The implication: building a new behavior and building a new identity are not sequential tasks. You don't wait until you've proven you're a person who exercises before you start describing yourself that way. You claim the identity slightly ahead of the evidence, and then let the identity pull the behavior into alignment. Each rep of the behavior becomes evidence for the identity. Each piece of evidence makes the next rep more likely. The loop reinforces itself in both directions.

This is why each chapter ends with "Becoming You" rather than "Maintaining Your New Habit." The goal is not a sustained effort of will. It's a shift in self-concept — from someone trying to do the thing, to someone who simply does it. That shift is the whole game.

Implementation Intentions

Where you'll find it: Every action step in every chapter

An implementation intention is a specific form of commitment that research consistently shows is more effective at producing behavior change than motivation, willpower, or general good intentions alone.

The format is: "When [situation X] occurs, I will do [behavior Y]." In the form used throughout this book: "Immediately after I [existing habit], I will [new behavior]."

The difference between "I'm going to exercise more" and "Immediately after I pour my morning coffee, I will do ten squats" is not cosmetic. It's architectural. The general intention leaves the decision to be made again under whatever conditions happen to exist at the moment of performance. The implementation intention removes the decision. The trigger fires. The behavior follows. System 1 stops arguing because there is nothing left to argue about.

Psychologist Peter Gollwitzer, who formalized the research basis for implementation intentions in 1999, found that people who specified when, where, and how they would perform a new behavior were two to three times more likely to follow through than people who only expressed the intention to do so. A meta-analysis of 94 independent studies confirmed the effect. The specificity isn't busywork. It's the mechanism.

Every fill-in-the-blank prompt in this book that begins with "Immediately after I _______, I will _______" is an implementation intention. The more specific the trigger and the behavior, the more likely the behavior is to happen.

Neuroplasticity

Where you'll find it: Introduction, throughout

Neuroplasticity is the brain's capacity to reorganize its structure, function, and connections in response to experience, learning, behavior, and environment. It is the neurobiological foundation on which this entire book rests.

For most of the twentieth century, the prevailing view was that the adult brain was essentially fixed: the neurons you had at birth were the neurons you'd always have, and the connections between them were largely set by early childhood. This view was wrong. Beginning in the 1970s and accelerating through the 1990s and 2000s, research demonstrated that the adult brain retains a substantial capacity for structural and functional change throughout the lifespan.

The mechanism follows Hebb's postulate, established in 1949 and now among the most replicated findings in neuroscience: neurons that fire together wire together, and neurons that stop firing together lose their connection. Repeated activation of a neural pathway strengthens it — the synapse becomes more efficient, the signal travels faster, the behavior becomes more automatic. Disuse has the opposite effect: pathways that go unactivated weaken and eventually prune.

This means that every behavior you repeat — including the ones you'd prefer to stop — is literally building structure in your brain. The pattern of anxiety that fires before social situations, the impulse to reach for the phone, the loop of self-critical thought that runs when you make a mistake — these are not character flaws. They are neural pathways that have been practiced, often thousands of times, and are now highly efficient. System 1 runs them.

The same mechanism that built those pathways can update them. It requires repetition, specificity, and time. It also requires conditions that support neuroplasticity — adequate sleep, regular movement, BDNF-promoting behaviors, and, in some cases, interventions like ketamine that create an enhanced neuroplastic window. The ten non-negotiables are, among other things, the conditions under which neuroplastic change becomes possible and durable.

The Rule of 60

Where you'll find it: Introduction, referenced throughout

The Rule of 60 comes from aviation navigation: for every one degree a plane drifts off its intended course, it will miss its destination by one mile for every sixty miles flown. On a short flight, one degree is noise. On a transcontinental flight, one degree is a different city.

In the Introduction, the Rule of 60 is used to explain how small, incremental neglect in any of the ten non-negotiables compounds into significant consequences over time. A sleep schedule that slips thirty minutes. A week without meaningful social contact. A month of meals that arrive in cardboard boxes. None of these feel like major decisions. The math catches up anyway.

As a planning tool, use it like this:

When you're considering a compromise — sleeping less than you planned, skipping a connection, letting a practice slip — ask: "if I make this same choice every day for sixty days, where does that put me? Is this a temporary, bounded deviation with a clear end point, or is this the beginning of a drift I won't notice until I've traveled a long way in the wrong direction?" Most self-defeating patterns don't begin with a dramatic decision. They begin with a degree.

The Rule of 60 works identically in the positive direction. One degree of consistent effort — a single small practice repeated daily — compounds with the same fidelity as neglect. This is why the book insists on starting small rather than starting impressively: small is what you'll maintain, and maintenance is what compounds. The goal is not a heroic first week. The goal is a degree you can hold for sixty.

The Small Self Response

Where you'll find it: Joy, Play & Awe, Meaning & Purpose (new nature insertion)

The small self response is a term from Dacher Keltner's research on awe at the University of California, Berkeley, describing the characteristic shift in self-perception that occurs during awe experiences.

Awe is the emotional response to encountering something vast, complex, or incomprehensible — something that exceeds your current mental frameworks and requires you to update them. The classic awe triggers are natural grandeur (a night sky, an ocean, a forest of old trees), music that opens something unexpected in the chest, witnessing extraordinary human achievement, or coming face to face with profound suffering or beauty in another person. What these experiences have in common is that they briefly dwarf the ordinary preoccupations of the self.

The small self response is what happens in that moment: the default mode network — the brain's self-referential processing system, responsible for the ongoing narrative of "I" — quiets. The internal monologue that runs almost continuously, assessing, comparing, planning, and worrying, pauses. In its place, there is a sense of being part of something larger. Keltner's research finds that this state is associated with reduced self-reported stress, increased feelings of meaning and connection, greater generosity toward others, and measurably lower levels of pro-inflammatory cytokines — the same inflammatory markers elevated in depression and PTSD.

The small self is not small in a diminishing sense. It is small in the way that being part of a vast whole is small — a reduction in the relentless centrality of personal concerns that, paradoxically, increases rather than diminishes the sense that one's existence matters.

Natural environments are among the most reliable and accessible triggers for this response. The research threshold is lower than most people assume: you do not need a mountain or an ocean. You need something genuinely vast or intricate that you slow down long enough to actually see — a cloud formation, a spider web, the particular quality of winter light, the fact that the soil under your feet contains more organisms than there are humans on the planet.

System 1 and System 2

Where you'll find it: Introduction, throughout

System 1 and System 2 are the two operating modes of the human mind, described by Nobel laureate Daniel Kahneman in his 2011 book Thinking, Fast and Slow, drawing on research by Keith Stanovich and Richard West.

System 1 is fast, automatic, and effortless. It runs below the level of conscious deliberation. It drives a familiar route without thinking, flinches before the threat has been consciously registered, reaches for the phone before a decision has been made. System 1 runs on pattern recognition, learned associations, and habit. Most of your behavior — the vast majority of what you actually do throughout a day — is run by System 1. It is not stupid or inferior. It is extraordinarily efficient, deeply adaptive, and essential for navigating a complex world without cognitive paralysis. The problem is that it faithfully runs whatever patterns it has learned, regardless of whether those patterns are serving you.

System 2 is slow, deliberate, and effortful. It does long division. It weighs a difficult decision. It notices that you've been scrolling for forty minutes. It can override System 1 — but it is expensive to run and cannot be sustained indefinitely. Depletion of System 2's resources (through fatigue, decision fatigue, or chronic stress) leaves System 1 in increasing control.

The relationship between the two systems is the central dynamic of behavior change. New skills begin in System 2: they require conscious effort, deliberate attention, and active decision-making. With repetition, they are gradually handed off to System 1, where they run automatically and efficiently. This handoff is neuroplasticity in action. The goal of the Four Drivers — and of every practice in this book — is to accelerate and support that handoff: to get the behaviors you want to choose into System 1, where they no longer require a decision.

This also explains why willpower is an unreliable strategy for long-term behavior change. Willpower is a System 2 function. It depletes. Environmental design, habit stacking, and identity-based framing are System 1 strategies — they work with the architecture of automaticity rather than fighting it.

Temptation Bundling

Where you'll find it: Movement, Life Administration — the "Link Habits" sections

Temptation bundling is the practice of pairing a behavior you want to build with an experience you genuinely enjoy — making the new behavior the condition of access to the pleasurable one.

The classic example from the Movement chapter: "I only listen to this podcast when I'm moving." The podcast is already rewarding to System 1. Movement is not yet. By making movement the price of admission for the podcast, you're not forcing yourself to exercise — you're making System 1 do the arithmetic and conclude that movement is worth it.

Behavioral economist Katy Milkman, who developed the formal research basis for temptation bundling, found that people who linked a "want" (something intrinsically enjoyable) to a "should" (something beneficial but not immediately rewarding) were significantly more likely to follow through with the "should" — and, crucially, to look forward to it rather than dread it. The motivational effect is durable: System 1 begins to associate the effortful behavior with the reward, which over time reduces the effort the behavior requires.

The design rules:

The enjoyable experience must be genuinely pleasurable — not merely neutral. The bundling must be strict: you only get the enjoyable experience when doing the target behavior. The exclusivity is what creates the leverage. And the enjoyable experience must be something you would otherwise want anyway — a podcast you're genuinely invested in, a coffee you'd drink regardless, a show you actually like.

Potential bundles across the ten non-negotiables:

- A favorite podcast or audiobook → only during walks, workouts, or outdoor movement
- An engaging audiobook → only during administrative tasks
- A specific tea or coffee ritual → only during your morning reflection or journaling time
- A show you're watching → only while doing light environmental maintenance
- A phone call with someone you enjoy → only during outdoor walks

The goal is not to bribe yourself. It's to design conditions under which System 1 stops resisting and starts cooperating.

Window of Tolerance

Where you'll find it: Self-Care, Physical Environment

The window of tolerance is the range of nervous system activation within which your brain can function at its best — processing information accurately, regulating emotion effectively, making decisions that reflect your values, and maintaining the cognitive flexibility that difficult situations require.

The concept was developed by psychiatrist and neuroscientist Daniel Siegel, building on earlier trauma research, and is now foundational in trauma-informed clinical work. Within the window, both brain systems are available: System 2 can think clearly, weigh options, and respond rather than react; System 1 is running efficiently without overwhelming the system with threat signals.

Outside the window, in either direction, the capacity for these functions degrades.

Hyperarousal — the upper edge of the window — is characterized by anxiety, panic, hypervigilance, anger, impulsivity, and intrusive thoughts. System 1 is running the threat response at high volume. System 2 is struggling to be heard.

Hypoarousal — the lower edge — is characterized by numbness, dissociation, collapse, shame, and the particular flatness of depression. The system has moved from mobilization to shutdown.

Both states are adaptive responses to perceived threat. Neither is a character flaw. Both become problematic when they are chronic — when the window is so narrowed by accumulated stress, trauma, or unmet basic needs that almost any demand pushes you outside it.

The goal of self-care, as described in this book, is not the elimination of stress. It is the widening of the window — expanding the range of conditions under which you can remain functional, responsive, and capable of choice. Sleep, movement, nature contact, regulation practices, and a supportive physical environment all contribute to a wider window. Chronic neglect of these inputs narrows it. The window is not fixed. It is responsive to what you put into the system.

Notes

1. The principle that repeated neural firing strengthens synaptic connections derives from Donald Hebb's foundational work: Hebb, D.O. (1949). *The Organization of Behavior: A Neuropsychological Theory.* Wiley. The popular shorthand "neurons that fire together wire together" is attributed to neuroscientist Carla Shatz as a summary of Hebb's postulate. For a contemporary treatment of synaptic plasticity, see: Kandel, E.R., Schwartz, J.H., Jessell, T.M., Siegelbaum, S.A., & Hudspeth, A.J. (2012). *Principles of Neural Science* (5th ed.). McGraw-Hill.

2. Kahneman, D. (2011). *Thinking, Fast and Slow.* Farrar, Straus and Giroux. The System 1/System 2 terminology was originally proposed by Stanovich, K.E., & West, R.F. (2000). Individual differences in reasoning: Implications for the rationality debate. *Behavioral and Brain Sciences, 23*(5), 645–665. Kahneman adopted and popularized the framework.

3. Kahneman (2011), p. 13. Kahneman writes: "The automatic operations of System 1 generate surprisingly complex patterns of ideas, but only the slower System 2 can construct thoughts in an orderly series of steps."

4. Implementation intentions were formalized by: Gollwitzer, P.M. (1999). Implementation intentions: Strong effects of simple plans. *American Psychologist, 54*(7), 493–503. The "after I X, I will Y" structure is the standard format. For application to habit formation: Fogg, B.J. (2020). *Tiny Habits: The Small Changes That Change Everything.* Houghton Mifflin Harcourt.

5. Fogg, B.J. (2020). *Tiny Habits*, pp. 51–78. Houghton Mifflin Harcourt. For the underlying dopaminergic reward mechanism: Schultz, W. (1998). Predictive reward signal of dopamine neurons. *Journal of Neurophysiology, 80*(1), 1–27.

6. Fogg, B.J. (2020). *Tiny Habits: The Small Changes That Change Everything.* Houghton Mifflin Harcourt. Clear, J. (2018). *Atomic Habits: Tiny Changes, Remarkable Results.* Avery/Penguin Random House. Both authors independently converge on the same core principles — small starting behaviors, environmental design, habit anchoring, and immediate reinforcement — drawing on overlapping bodies of behavioral science research.

7. Gollwitzer, P.M. (1999). Implementation intentions: Strong effects of simple plans. *American Psychologist,* 54(7), 493–503. A meta-analysis of 94 independent tests found that implementation intentions had a medium-to-large effect on goal achievement compared to goal intentions alone. Gollwitzer, P.M., & Sheeran, P. (2006). Implementation intentions and goal achievement: A meta-analysis of effects and processes. *Advances in Experimental Social Psychology,* 38, 69–119.

8. The glymphatic system and its role in clearing metabolic waste during sleep was described in: Iliff, J.J., Wang, M., Liao, Y., Plogg, B.A., Peng, W., Gundersen, G.A., ... & Nedergaard, M. (2012). A paravascular pathway facilitates CSF flow through the brain parenchyma and the clearance of interstitial solutes, including amyloid β. *Science Translational Medicine,* 4(147), 147ra111. For a broader treatment: Walker, M. (2017). *Why We Sleep: Unlocking the Power of Sleep and Dreams.* Scribner.

9. The two-process model of sleep regulation — circadian rhythm and homeostatic sleep drive — was established by: Borbély, A.A. (1982). A two process model of sleep regulation. *Human Neurobiology, 1*(3), 195–204. For a comprehensive review: Dijk, D.J., & Lockley, S.W. (2002). Invited review: Integration of human

sleep-wake regulation and circadian rhythmicity. *Journal of Applied Physiology*, 92(2), 852–862.

10. Adenosine accumulation as the mechanism of homeostatic sleep drive: Porkka-Heiskanen, T., Strecker, R.E., Thakkar, M., Bjørkum, A.A., Greene, R.W., & McCarley, R.W. (1997). Adenosine: A mediator of the sleep-inducing effects of prolonged wakefulness. *Science*, *276*(5316), 1265–1268.

11. Caffeine's mechanism of action as an adenosine receptor antagonist: Fredholm, B.B., Bättig, K., Holmén, J., Nehlig, A., & Zvartau, E.E. (1999). Actions of caffeine in the brain with special reference to factors that contribute to its widespread use. *Pharmacological Reviews*, *51*(1), 83–133.

12. Sleep architecture and 90-minute ultradian cycles: Carskadon, M.A., & Dement, W.C. (2005). Normal human sleep: An overview. In M.H. Kryger, T. Roth, & W.C. Dement (Eds.), *Principles and Practice of Sleep Medicine* (4th ed., pp. 13–23). Elsevier. For accessible treatment: Walker, M. (2017). *Why We Sleep*. Scribner.

13. The equivalence of 24-hour sleep deprivation to 0.10% blood-alcohol impairment: Williamson, A.M., & Feyer, A.M. (2000). Moderate sleep deprivation produces impairments in cognitive and motor performance equivalent to legally prescribed levels of alcohol intoxication. *Occupational and Environmental Medicine*, 57(10), 649–655.

14. Memory consolidation during non-REM sleep and emotional processing during REM: Walker, M.P., & Stickgold, R. (2004). Sleep-dependent learning and memory consolidation. *Neuron*, 44(1), 121–133. For emotional processing: Walker, M.P., & van der Helm, E. (2009). Overnight therapy? The role of sleep in emotional brain processing. *Psychological Bulletin*, *135*(5), 731–748.

15. The bidirectional relationship between sleep and mood disorders: Baglioni, C., Battagliese, G., Feige, B., Spiegelhalder, K., Nissen, C.,

Voderholzer, U., ... & Riemann, D. (2011). Insomnia as a predictor of depression: A meta-analytic evaluation of longitudinal epidemiological studies. *Journal of Affective Disorders, 135*(1–3), 10–19.

16. BDNF and its role in neuroplasticity is detailed in: Ratey, J.J., & Hagerman, E. (2008). *Spark: The Revolutionary New Science of Exercise and the Brain.* Little, Brown. Note: the "Miracle-Gro for the brain" phrase is Ratey's coinage, not Sapolsky's. For the primary research: Cotman, C.W., & Berchtold, N.C. (2002). Exercise: A behavioral intervention to enhance brain health and plasticity. *Trends in Neurosciences, 25*(6), 295–301.

17. Exercise and prefrontal cortex blood flow and function: Colcombe, S.J., Kramer, A.F., Erickson, K.I., Scalf, P., McAuley, E., Cohen, N.J., ... & Elavsky, S. (2004). Cardiovascular fitness, cortical plasticity, and aging. *Proceedings of the National Academy of Sciences, 101*(9), 3316–3321.

18. Strength training and executive function: Liu-Ambrose, T., Nagamatsu, L.S., Graf, P., Beattie, B.L., Ashe, M.C., & Handy, T.C. (2010). Resistance training and executive functions: A 12-month randomized controlled trial. *Archives of Internal Medicine, 170*(2), 170–178.

19. Yoga, tai chi, cortisol regulation and mood: Pascoe, M.C., Thompson, D.R., Jenkins, Z.M., & Ski, C.F. (2017). Mindfulness mediates the physiological markers of stress: Systematic review and meta-analysis. *Journal of Psychiatric Research, 95*, 156–178.

20. Exercise as an evidence-based intervention for depression and anxiety: Blumenthal, J.A., Babyak, M.A., Moore, K.A., Craighead, W.E., Herman, S., Khatri, P., ... & Krishnan, K.R. (1999). Effects of exercise training on older patients with major depression. *Archives of Internal Medicine, 159*(19), 2349–2356. For a comprehensive review: Craft, L.L., & Perna, F.M. (2004). The benefits of exercise for the

clinically depressed. *Primary Care Companion to the Journal of Clinical Psychiatry*, 6(3), 104–111.

21. Brain fat composition and myelin: Chang, C.Y., Ke, D.S., & Chen, J.Y. (2009). Essential fatty acids and human brain. *Acta Neurologica Taiwanica*, *18*(4), 231–241.

22. Brain water content: Wenger, C.B. (2005). Human adaptations to hot climates. In K.B. Pandolf & R.E. Burr (Eds.), *Medical Aspects of Harsh Environments* (Vol. 1). Borden Institute. The 73% figure is established in: Bhagat, R.K. (2013). Water content of the brain. *Human Physiology*, 39(6).

23. Dehydration and cognitive impairment at 2% body water loss: Ganio, M.S., Armstrong, L.E., Casa, D.J., McDermott, B.P., Lee, E.C., Yamamoto, L.M., ... & Lieberman, H.R. (2011). Mild dehydration impairs cognitive performance and mood of men. *British Journal of Nutrition*, *106*(10), 1535–1543. Also: Adan, A. (2012). Cognitive performance and dehydration. *Journal of the American College of Nutrition*, *31*(2), 71–78.

24. Gut serotonin production: Yano, J.M., Yu, K., Donaldson, G.P., Shastri, G.G., Ann, P., Ma, L., ... & Hsiao, E.Y. (2015). Indigenous bacteria from the gut microbiota regulate host serotonin biosynthesis. *Cell*, *161*(2), 264–276. The 90% figure is widely cited; for context: Gershon, M.D. (1998). *The Second Brain.* HarperCollins.

25. Inflammation as a correlate of depression and cytokine-mediated serotonin impairment: Dantzer, R., O'Connor, J.C., Freund, G.G., Johnson, R.W., & Kelley, K.W. (2008). From inflammation to sickness and depression: When the immune system subjugates the brain. *Nature Reviews Neuroscience*, 9(1), 46–56. Also: Miller, A.H., Maletic, V., & Raison, C.L. (2009). Inflammation and its discontents: The role of cytokines in the pathophysiology of major depression. *Biological Psychiatry*, 65(9), 732–741.

26. The window of tolerance concept was developed by: Siegel, D.J. (1999). *The Developing Mind: How Relationships and the Brain Interact to Shape Who We Are.* Guilford Press. Further elaborated in: Ogden, P., Minton, K., & Pain, C. (2006). *Trauma and the Body: A Sensorimotor Approach to Psychotherapy.* Norton.

27. Prefrontal cortex impairment under chronic stress: Arnsten, A.F.T. (2009). Stress signalling pathways that impair prefrontal cortex structure and function. *Nature Reviews Neuroscience, 10*(6), 410–422. Also: McEwen, B.S., & Morrison, J.H. (2013). The brain on stress: Vulnerability and plasticity of the prefrontal cortex over the life course. *Neuron,* 79(1), 16–29.

28. Environmental stressors, HPA axis activation, and cortisol: Evans, G.W. (2006). Child development and the physical environment. *Annual Review of Psychology, 57,* 423–451. For noise specifically: Stansfeld, S.A., & Matheson, M.P. (2003). Noise pollution: Non-auditory effects on health. *British Medical Bulletin, 68*(1), 243–257.

29. Allostatic load as cumulative biological wear from chronic stress: McEwen, B.S., & Stellar, E. (1993). Stress and the individual: Mechanisms leading to disease. *Archives of Internal Medicine, 153*(18), 2093–2101. For the full concept: McEwen, B.S. (1998). Stress, adaptation, and disease: Allostasis and allostatic load. *Annals of the New York Academy of Sciences, 840,* 33–44.

30. Restorative environments and stress marker reduction: Ulrich, R.S., Simons, R.F., Losito, B.D., Fiorito, E., Miles, M.A., & Zelson, M. (1991). Stress recovery during exposure to natural and urban environments. *Journal of Environmental Psychology, 11*(3), 201–230. Also: Kaplan, R., & Kaplan, S. (1989). *The Experience of Nature: A Psychological Perspective.* Cambridge University Press.

31. Decision fatigue — the depletion of decision-making quality over multiple decisions: Baumeister, R.F., Bratslavsky, E., Muraven, M., & Tice, D.M. (1998). Ego depletion: Is the active self a limited resource?

Journal of Personality and Social Psychology, 74(5), 1252–1265. For applied research: Danziger, S., Levav, J., & Avnaim-Pesso, L. (2011). Extraneous factors in judicial decisions. *Proceedings of the National Academy of Sciences, 108*(17), 6889–6892.

32. The "15 cigarettes a day" mortality comparison is not Cacioppo's original finding but derives from: Holt-Lunstad, J., Smith, T.B., & Layton, J.B. (2010). Social relationships and mortality risk: A meta-analytic review. *PLOS Medicine*, 7(7), e1000316. Also: Holt-Lunstad, J., Smith, T.B., Baker, M., Harris, T., & Stephenson, D. (2015). Loneliness and social isolation as risk factors for mortality: A meta-analytic review. *Perspectives on Psychological Science, 10*(2), 227–237. Cacioppo's foundational loneliness research is: Cacioppo, J.T., & Patrick, W. (2008). *Loneliness: Human Nature and the Need for Social Connection.* Norton.

33. Oxytocin, amygdala reactivity, and social stress response: Heinrichs, M., Baumgartner, T., Kirschbaum, C., & Ehlert, U. (2003). Social support and oxytocin interact to suppress cortisol and subjective responses to psychosocial stress. *Biological Psychiatry,* 54(12), 1389–1398.

34. Loneliness, hypervigilance, and hostile attribution bias: Cacioppo, J.T., Hawkley, L.C., & Berntson, G.G. (2003). The anatomy of loneliness. *Current Directions in Psychological Science, 12*(3), 71–74. Also: Cacioppo, J.T., & Hawkley, L.C. (2009). Perceived social isolation and cognition. *Trends in Cognitive Sciences, 13*(10), 447–454.

35. Frankl, V.E. (1946/2006). *Man's Search for Meaning.* Beacon Press. Originally published in German in 1946; the standard English edition is the 2006 Beacon Press paperback. For logotherapy's clinical framework: Frankl, V.E. (1967). *Psychotherapy and Existentialism: Selected Papers on Logotherapy.* Simon & Schuster.

36. Values alignment and intrinsic versus extrinsic dopaminergic motivation: Ryan, R.M., & Deci, E.L. (2000). Self-determination

theory and the facilitation of intrinsic motivation, social development, and well-being. *American Psychologist*, *55*(1), 68–78. For neurobiological underpinning: Murayama, K., Matsumoto, M., Izuma, K., & Matsumoto, K. (2010). Neural basis of the undermining effect of extrinsic reward on intrinsic motivation. *Proceedings of the National Academy of Sciences*, *107*(49), 20911–20916.

37. Meaning-making as a component of PTSD treatment: Park, C.L. (2010). Making sense of the meaning literature: An integrative review of meaning making and its effects on adjustment to stressful life events. *Psychological Bulletin*, *136*(2), 257–301. For narrative integration specifically: Pennebaker, J.W., & Beall, S.K. (1986). Confronting a traumatic event: Toward an understanding of inhibition and disease. *Journal of Abnormal Psychology*, *95*(3), 274–281.

38. Prosocial behavior, dopamine, and oxytocin reward pathways: Moll, J., Krueger, F., Zahn, R., Pardini, M., de Oliveira-Souza, R., & Grafman, J. (2006). Human fronto-mesolimbic networks guide decisions about charitable donation. *Proceedings of the National Academy of Sciences*, *103*(42), 15623–15628. For oxytocin specifically: Zak, P.J., Stanton, A.A., & Ahmadi, S. (2007). Oxytocin increases generosity in humans. *PLOS ONE*, *2*(11), e1128.

39. Default mode network activity and self-referential processing in depression: Sheline, Y.I., Barch, D.M., Price, J.L., Rundle, M.M., Vaishnavi, S.N., Snyder, A.Z., ... & Raichle, M.E. (2009). The default mode network and self-referential processes in depression. *Proceedings of the National Academy of Sciences*, *106*(6), 1942–1947.

40. Fredrickson, B.L. (2001). The role of positive emotions in positive psychology: The broaden-and-build theory of positive emotions. *American Psychologist*, *56*(3), 218–226. Also: Fredrickson, B.L. (2004). The broaden-and-build theory of positive emotions. *Philosophical Transactions of the Royal Society B*, *359*(1449), 1367–1377.

41. Brown, S., & Vaughan, C. (2009). *Play: How It Shapes the Brain, Opens the Imagination, and Invigorates the Soul.* Avery/Penguin. Brown's research on play deprivation is summarized throughout; for academic grounding see also: Pellegrini, A.D., & Smith, P.K. (1998). Physical activity play: The nature and function of a neglected aspect of play. *Child Development, 69*(3), 577–598.

42. Keltner's research on awe and inflammatory cytokines: Stellar, J.E., John-Henderson, N., Anderson, C.L., Gordon, A.M., McNeil, G.D., & Keltner, D. (2015). Positive affect and markers of inflammation: Discrete positive emotions predict lower levels of inflammatory cytokines. *Emotion, 15*(2), 129–133. For the broader awe research program: Keltner, D., & Haidt, J. (2003). Approaching awe, a moral, spiritual, and aesthetic emotion. *Cognition and Emotion, 17*(2), 297–314.

43. Time Americans spend indoors: Klepeis, N.E., Nelson, W.C., Ott, W.R., Robinson, J.P., Tsang, A.M., Switzer, P., ... & Engelmann, W.H. (2001). The National Human Activity Pattern Survey (NHAPS): A resource for assessing exposure to environmental pollutants. *Journal of Exposure Analysis and Environmental Epidemiology, 11*(3), 231–252. The 90 percent figure is the widely cited summary statistic from this EPA-funded survey of 9,386 respondents.

44. Cortisol reduction, blood pressure reduction, and autonomic recovery in natural versus built environments: Ulrich, R.S., Simons, R.F., Losito, B.D., Fiorito, E., Miles, M.A., & Zelson, M. (1991). Stress recovery during exposure to natural and urban environments. *Journal of Environmental Psychology, 11*(3), 201–230. Also: Kaplan, R., & Kaplan, S. (1989). *The Experience of Nature: A Psychological Perspective.* Cambridge University Press. For a meta-analytic synthesis: Bowler, D.E., Buyung-Ali, L.M., Knight, T.M., & Pullin, A.S. (2010). A systematic review of evidence for the added benefits to health of exposure to natural environments. *BMC Public Health, 10,* 456.

45. Morning natural light exposure and circadian anchoring: Wright, K.P., McHill, A.W., Birks, B.R., Griffin, B.R., Rusterholz, T., & Czeisler, C.A. (2013). Entrainment of the human circadian clock to the natural light-dark cycle. *Current Biology, 23*(16), 1554–1558. For the downstream effects on sleep architecture and mood: Leproult, R., Colecchia, E.F., L'Hermite-Balériaux, M., & Van Cauter, E. (2001). Transition from dim to bright light in the morning induces an immediate elevation of cortisol levels. *Journal of Clinical Endocrinology & Metabolism, 86*(1), 151–157.

46. Microbiome diversity and contact with natural environments and soil: Rook, G.A.W. (2013). Regulation of the immune system by biodiversity from the natural environment: An ecosystem service essential to health. *Proceedings of the National Academy of Sciences, 110*(46), 18360–18367. Also: Flies, E.J., Skelly, C., Negi, S.S., Prabhala, P., Singh, R., Hocking, D., ... & Weinstein, P. (2017). Biodiverse green spaces: A prescription for global urban health. *Frontiers in Ecology and the Environment, 15*(9), 510–516.

47. Parasympathetic activation in natural environments: Park, B.J., Tsunetsugu, Y., Kasetani, T., Kagawa, T., & Miyazaki, Y. (2010). The physiological effects of Shinrin-yoku (taking in the forest atmosphere or forest bathing): Evidence from field experiments in 24 forests across Japan. *Environmental Health and Preventive Medicine, 15*(1), 18–26. For the autonomic nervous system mechanism specifically: Gladwell, V.F., Brown, D.K., Wood, C., Sandercock, G.R., & Barton, J. (2013). The great outdoors: How a green exercise environment can benefit all. *Extreme Physiology & Medicine*, 2(1), 3.

48. Suprachiasmatic nucleus, morning light intensity, and circadian clock setting: Reppert, S.M., & Weaver, D.R. (2002). Coordination of circadian timing in mammals. *Nature, 418*(6901), 935–941. For light intensity thresholds and SCN sensitivity: Zeitzer, J.M., Dijk, D.J., Kronauer, R., Brown, E., & Czeisler, C. (2000). Sensitivity of the human circadian pacemaker to nocturnal light: Melatonin phase resetting and suppression. *Journal of Physiology*, 526(3), 695–702.

Outdoor daylight (even overcast) typically ranges from 1,000 to 10,000 lux; standard indoor lighting is 100–500 lux.

49. Outdoor versus indoor exercise — cortisol, mood, perceived exertion, and intention to repeat: Coon, J.T., Boddy, K., Stein, K., Whear, R., Barton, J., & Depledge, M.H. (2011). Does participating in physical activity in outdoor natural environments have a greater effect on physical and mental wellbeing than physical activity indoors? A systematic review. *Environmental Science & Technology, 45*(5), 1761–1772. Also: Ekkekakis, P., Parfitt, G., & Petruzzello, S.J. (2011). The pleasure and displeasure people feel when they exercise at different intensities. *Sports Medicine, 41*(8), 641–671.

50. Shinrin-yoku / forest bathing research — cortisol, blood pressure, natural killer cell activity, and phytoncides: Li, Q., Morimoto, K., Nakadai, A., Inagaki, H., Katsumata, M., Shimizu, T., ... & Kawada, T. (2007). Forest bathing enhances human natural killer activity and expression of anti-cancer proteins. *International Journal of Immunopathology and Pharmacology, 20*(2 Suppl 2), 3–8. For the phytoncide mechanism specifically: Li, Q., Nakadai, A., Matsushima, H., Miyazaki, Y., Blumenfield, A.M., Krensky, A.M., & Kawada, T. (2006). Phytoncides (wood essential oils) induce human natural killer cell activity. *Immunopharmacology and Immunotoxicology, 28*(2), 319–333. For the comprehensive review: Li, Q. (2010). Effect of forest bathing trips on human immune function. *Environmental Health and Preventive Medicine, 15*(1), 9–17.

51. Twenty minutes in natural settings two to three times per week and sustained cortisol reduction: Hunter, M.R., Gillespie, B.W., & Chen, S.Y. (2019). Urban nature experiences reduce stress in the context of daily life based on salivary biomarkers. *Frontiers in Psychology, 10*, 722. This study found that 20–30 minutes of nature contact produced the steepest cortisol reduction curves, with benefits plateauing at approximately 200 minutes. Frequency of two to three sessions per week was sufficient to sustain reduced baseline cortisol over the measurement period.

52. Forty-second green micro-exposure restoring attention and reducing error rates: Lee, K.E., Williams, K.J.H., Sargent, L.D., Williams, N.S.G., & Johnson, K.A. (2015). 40-second green roof views sustain attention: The role of micro-breaks in attention restoration. *Journal of Environmental Psychology*, 42, 182–189. Participants performed a sustained-attention task and those given a 40-second break with a view of a green rooftop showed significantly better performance and fewer errors in the subsequent task than those given an equivalent break with a view of a concrete rooftop.

53. Attention Restoration Theory — involuntary attention, directed attention fatigue, and restoration in natural environments: Kaplan, S. (1995). The restorative benefits of nature: Toward an integrative framework. *Journal of Environmental Psychology*, *15*(3), 169–182. The foundational theoretical paper distinguishing directed and involuntary attention and establishing natural environments as preferentially restorative. Also: Kaplan, R., & Kaplan, S. (1989). *The Experience of Nature: A Psychological Perspective.* Cambridge University Press. For empirical support: Berman, M.G., Jonides, J., & Kaplan, S. (2008). The cognitive benefits of interacting with nature. *Psychological Science*, *19*(12), 1207–1212.

54. Ulrich's 1984 hospital window study: Ulrich, R.S. (1984). View through a window may influence recovery from surgery. *Science*, 224(4647), 420–421. Patients recovering from cholecystectomy whose windows faced a stand of trees had shorter post-surgical hospital stays, received fewer negative evaluative comments from nurses, required less pain medication, and had lower complication rates than matched patients whose windows faced a brick wall.

55. Indoor plants and effects on air quality, attention, and stress perception: Bringslimark, T., Hartig, T., & Patil, G.G. (2009). The psychological benefits of indoor plants: A critical review of the experimental literature. *Journal of Environmental Psychology*, 29(4), 422–433. Also: Lohr, V.I., Pearson-Mims, C.H., & Goodwin, G.K. (1996). Interior plants may improve worker productivity and reduce

stress in a windowless environment. *Journal of Environmental Horticulture*, *14*(2), 97–100.

56. Outdoor side-by-side activity and social bonding: Johansson, M., Hartig, T., & Staats, H. (2011). Psychological benefits of walking: Moderation by company and outdoor environment. *Applied Psychology: Health and Well-Being*, *3*(3), 261–280. This study found that walking with a companion in a natural setting produced significantly greater improvements in mood, social bonding, and self-reported openness compared to walking with a companion in an urban environment. Also: Duvall, J. (2011). Enhancing the benefits of outdoor walking with cognitive engagement strategies. *Journal of Environmental Psychology*, *31*(1), 27–35. The "soft fascination" mechanism derives from Kaplan, S. (1995) — see note 53.

57. Soil biodiversity: Estimates of microbial diversity in one gram of soil have been placed at between 10,000 and 50,000 distinct species: Torsvik, V., Goksøyr, J., & Daae, F.L. (1990). High diversity in DNA of soil bacteria. *Applied and Environmental Microbiology*, *56*(3), 782–787. For the broader "more organisms per gram of soil than humans on Earth" framing: Kallmeyer, J., Pockalny, R., Adhikari, R.R., Smith, D.C., & D'Hondt, S. (2012). Global distribution of microbial abundance and biomass in subseafloor sediment. *Proceedings of the National Academy of Sciences*, *109*(40), 16213–16216.

About the Authors

Oli Mittermaier, MS

Oli Mittermaier is the co-founder of CIT Clinics, where he and Adam Tibble have treated patients in psychological distress over the past decade. He oversees patient care and program development, with a particular focus on what determines whether clinical treatment translates into long-term recovery.

A graduate of the University of Pennsylvania, Oli has spent his career at the intersection of leadership, mental health, and human performance. Before founding CIT Clinics, he facilitated emotional intelligence and leadership programs at Fortune 500 companies for many years. He is a certified Search Inside Yourself teacher (the mindfulness-based emotional intelligence program developed at Google), an instructor with the National Outdoor Leadership School (NOLS), and a TEDx speaker.

Born in Portugal to German parents and raised in Switzerland, Oli lives in Fairfax, California. He hosts a daily online practice community called 15 Minutes of Positivity.

Adam Tibble, MD

Adam Tibble is the co-founder and medical director of CIT Clinics. A board-certified anesthesiologist, he is responsible for the clinical protocols and medical oversight of every ketamine-assisted treatment at CIT Clinics.

A veteran of the United States Air Force, Adam served two combat deployments to Afghanistan with the Critical Care Air Transport Team (CCATT) — one of the most demanding clinical roles in modern military medicine. CCATT physicians stabilize and transport severely wounded patients on long-distance flights, managing the most acute presentations of physical trauma, neurological injury, and psychological distress in austere conditions, often simultaneously.

That experience shaped his understanding of what it takes to keep a person alive during acute crisis — and what comes after the crisis has passed.

Adam lives in Davis, California.

www.ingramcontent.com/pod-product-compliance
Lightning Source LLC
LaVergne TN
LVHW100521110826
845146LV00002B/725

* 9 7 9 8 9 9 6 1 1 7 3 0 7 *